Invariant Measurement

This introductory text describes the principles of invariant measurement, how invariant measurement can be achieved with Rasch models, and how to use invariant measurement to solve measurement problems in the social, behavioral, and health sciences. Rasch models are used throughout but a comparison of Rasch models to other item response theory (IRT) models is also provided.

Written with students in mind, the manuscript was class tested to help maximize accessibility. Chapters open with an introduction and close with a summary and discussion. Numerous examples and exercises demonstrate the main issues addressed in each chapter. Key terms are defined when first introduced and in an end-of-text glossary. All of the book's analyses were conducted with the Facets program. The data sets used in the book, sample syntax files for running the Facets program, Excel files for creating item and person response functions, links to related websites, and other material are available at www.GeorgeEngelhard.com.

Highlights include:
- A strong philosophical and methodological approach to measurement in the human sciences
- Demonstrations of how measurement problems can be addressed using invariant measurement
- Practical illustrations of how to create and evaluate scales using invariant measurement
- A history of measurement based on test-score and scaling traditions
- Previously unpublished work in analyzing rating data, the detection and measurement of rater errors, and the evaluation of rater accuracy
- A review of estimation methods, model-data fit, indices used to evaluate the quality of rater-mediated assessments, rater error and bias, and rater accuracy.

Intended as a supplementary text for graduate or advanced undergraduate courses on measurement or test theory, item response theory, scaling theory, psychometrics, advanced measurement techniques, research methods, or evaluation research taught in education, psychology, and the social and health sciences, the book also appeals to practitioners and researchers in these fields who develop or use scales and instruments. Only a basic mathematical level is required including a basic course in statistics.

George Engelhard, Jr. is Professor of Educational Measurement and Policy at Emory University. He received his Ph.D. from the University of Chicago, USA.

Invariant Measurement

Using Rasch Models in the Social, Behavioral, and Health Sciences

George Engelhard, Jr.

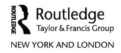

Routledge
Taylor & Francis Group

NEW YORK AND LONDON

First published 2013
by Routledge
711 Third Avenue, New York, NY 10017

Simultaneously published in the UK
by Routledge
27 Church Road, Hove, East Sussex BN3 2FA

Routledge is an imprint of the Taylor & Francis Group, an informa business

Library of Congress Cataloging in Publication Data
Engelhard, George, 1953–
    Invariant measurement : using Rasch models in the social, behavioral, and health sciences / by George Engelhard, Jr.
    p. cm.
    ISBN 978-0-415-87122-8 (hbk. : alk. paper) – ISBN 978-0-203-07363-6 (pbk. : alk. paper) 1. Psychometrics. 2. Invariant measures. 3. Rasch models. 4. Psychology–Statistical methods. 5. Social sciences—Statistical methods. I. Title.
    BF39.E54 2012
    150.28'7–dc23
    2012027583

ISBN: 978-0-415-87122-8 (hbk)
ISBN: 978-0-415-87125-9 (pbk)
ISBN: 978-0-203-07363-6 (ebk)

Typeset in Times New Roman
by EvS Communication Networx, Inc.

To Judy Monsaas, Emily Monsaas Engelhard, and
David Monsaas Engelhard ~ my love for you is invariant!

Contents

Preface

Aims of the Book

The major aims of this book are to describe in detail the principles of invariant measurement, to illustrate how invariant measurement can be achieved with Rasch measurement models, and to demonstrate the use of invariant measurement to solve measurement problems in the social, behavioral, and health sciences. This book was written to provide an introduction to the idea of Invariant Measurement. The book combines a descriptive and accessible introduction to Rasch measurement models with a strong underlying philosophy of measurement that undergirds the development and use of assessments in the human sciences.

Audiences for the Book

Invariant Measurement is intended for undergraduate and graduate students in the social, behavioral, and health sciences with an interest in measurement. It should also be of interest to measurement practitioners who work on the development of instruments and scales. This book is accessible to researchers in various fields who use rating scales and other judgmental procedures requiring rater-mediated assessments. The content of the book can form the basis for graduate seminars and courses on measurement in various disciplines including education, psychology, public health, nursing, sociology, applied linguistics, and political science. The book can also serve as an additional reading for advanced undergraduate and graduate courses in psychometrics and research methodology, item response theory, scaling theory, evaluation research, etc. This book can also be used independently by researchers interested in learning about invariant measurement and Rasch models.

The cognitive demand is moderately rigorous, but the content should be accessible to motivated undergraduate and graduate students with an interest in invariant measurement. The quantitative prerequisites are minimal. All of the numerical methods are described in enough detail so that only a basic mathematical level is required. For example, the text should be readily accessible to students who have completed an introductory course in statistics. I have used similar material over the past 15 years in graduate seminars at Emory University, Temple University Japan, and the National University of Singapore. These seminars have included students from various fields with very limited mathematical backgrounds. The major prerequisites are the ability to think logically, and the motivation to learn about invariant measurement.

Invariant Measurement is appropriate for the same audiences as *Applying the Rasch Model: Fundamental Measurement in the Human Sciences* (Bond & Fox, 2007), and *Constructing Measures: An Item Response Modeling Approach* (Wilson, 2005). I have used both of these excellent books in graduate seminars at Emory University over the past few years. The content of *Invariant Measurement: Using Rasch Models in the Social, Behavioral, and Health Sciences* complements these two books. It is easy to envision readers using this book in conjunction with these other two books on measurement. Of course, *Invariant Measurement* can stand alone as a separate contribution on measurement in the social, behavioral, and health sciences.

Overall Structure of the Book

The first four chapters provide an introduction to invariant measurement based on the Rasch model. The five requirements of invariant measurement are described in Chapter 1. Chapters 2 and 3 provide descriptions of item-invariant person measurement and person-invariant item calibration based on a family of Rasch measurement models (Dichotomous Model, Partial Credit Model, Rating Scale Model, and Many Facet Model). A detailed description of how to construct measures based on Wilson's (2005) approach is included in Chapter 4. Chapters 5 and 6 provide historical and comparative perspectives on the key ideas under girding invariant measurement. Chapter 7 covers a variety of estimation methods that researchers and theorists have proposed for estimating the parameters in Rasch models, while Chapter 8 introduces the important idea of model-data fit. Chapter 9 describes a conceptual framework that views raters and other aspects of rater-mediated assessments in terms of a lens model (Brunswik, 1952). The following two chapters describe an array of indices that can use to evaluate the quality of rater-mediated assessments using direct and indirect indicators of rater agreement, rater error and bias, and rater accuracy. The final chapter briefly addresses various topics related to perennial issues in assessment from the perspective of invariant measurement.

Getting Started (Learning Tools)

All of the analyses in this book were conducted with the Facets computer program (Linacre, 2007). Free student versions of this program are available online at www.winsteps.com. The data sets used in this book, sample syntax files for running the Facets computer program, Excel files for creating item and person response functions, links to key websites regarding advances in Rasch measurement theory, and other supportive material regarding invariant measurement are available at www.GeorgeEngelhard.com. I invite motivated readers to join the vibrant and strong community of scholars who work on the development of Rasch measurement theory, and who are actively involved in the quest for invariant measurement in the human sciences. A special version of the Facets computer program (IM_Facets) is available on the website for analyzing the data sets in the book.

Acknowledgments

In the fall of 1977, I started my Ph.D. program at the University of Chicago in measurement, evaluation, and statistical analysis (MESA Program). One summer day before my admission to the U of C, I had the great pleasure of meeting Professors Ben Bloom, Ben Wright. and R. Darrell Bock. After these meetings, I was convinced that the MESA Program was the place for me to finally figure out how to address the measurement problems that existed in the social sciences. My undergraduate major was in sociology, and, in one of my first courses on social science research methods, I encountered the work of Paul Lazarsfeld (Lazarsfeld, 1966; Lazarsfeld & Henry, 1968)—I was convinced that the only way to move forward in theory and practice in the social sciences was to address the persistent measurement problems. Adequate statistical models were clearly available, but insufficient attention had been paid to how to measure the key constructs and latent variables of interest. I have made the quest for high quality measurement in the social, behavioral, and health sciences the major theme in my professional life.

Ben Wright sent me home after our initial meeting with two articles: Wright (1968) and Choppin (1968). I have spent many years trying to fully understand the power and usefulness of Rasch models. The key concept that separates Rasch models from other test theories, such as classical test theory, is that under appropriate conditions it is possible to obtain invariant measurement. The essence of invariant measurement as I first encountered it in the summer of 1977 is embodied in this quote:

> First, the calibration of measuring instruments must be independent of those objects that happen to be used for calibration. Second, the measurement of objects must be independent of the instrument that happens to be used for the measuring. (Wright, 1968, p. 87)

The first part of this quote refers to sample-invariant item calibration, while the second part refers to item-invariant measurement of individuals. The basic measurement problem addressed by sample-invariant item calibration is how to minimize the influences of arbitrary samples of individuals on the estimation of item scale values or item difficulties. The overall goal of sample-invariant measurement can be viewed as estimating the locations of items on a latent variable or construct of interest that will remain unchanged across various subgroups of persons. In the case of item-invariant measurement, the basic measurement problem is to minimize the influence of the particular items that happen to be used to estimate a person's location on the latent variable or construct. Every yardstick and measuring instrument should yield comparable measures of an object's length regardless the particular yardstick or instrument used for the measurement process. Issues related to invariant measurement represent some of the fundamental problems in measurement theory.

Ben Bloom once pointed out to me that assessments can be viewed as a technology with great potential for good, and also for harm.

> It is no great exaggeration to compare the power of testing on human affairs with the power of atomic energy. Both are capable of great positive benefit to all of mankind and both contain equally great potential for destroying mankind. If mankind is to survive, we must continually search for the former and seek ways of controlling or limiting the later. (Bloom, 1970, p. 26)

After spending more than 30 years working in assessment and serving on numerous technical advisory committees at the state, national and international levels, it is now clear to me that there is much truth in Bloom's observation. I am also more convinced than ever that my insight as an undergraduate student regarding the importance of measurement was accurate and that measurement continues to be a critical issue in the social, behavioral, and health sciences to the present day.

In 1985, I joined the faculty at Emory University with appointments in the college and graduate school of arts and sciences. During my years at Emory University, I have taught educational measurement to undergraduate students, preservice teachers, and graduate students. I have also taught annual measurement seminars each spring on Rasch measurement, researcher-constructed measures, and the history of measurement theory. Recently, I have been lecturing at Temple University Japan and the National University of Singapore on issues related to the assessment of English as a second language, and on language assessment issues in general. I have learned much from my interactions with many students and colleagues over the years.

Much of the work in this book related to rater-mediated assessment began when I was first invited to work on the problem of developing a psychometrically defensible performance assessment of writing in Georgia. I have also been strongly influenced by my graduate students who have worked on various applications of Rasch measurement theory to topics including writing assessment, rater judgments, grading practices, and nursing practices. My debt to students in these seminars should be obvious in the pages of this book.

In 1986, I served on my first technical advisory committee in Georgia. My views have been deeply influenced by my attempts to put measurement theory into practice within the context of statewide assessments and accountability systems in educational settings. In every case, the use of Rasch models has increased our substantive and methodological understanding of a host of measurement problems. These problem areas include teacher assessments (National Board for Professional Teaching Standards), equating and linking issues, differential item and person functioning, rater-mediated assessments and standard setting. Colleagues and students have also greatly influenced my thinking and shaped my views of measurement. In particular, I would like to mention David Andrich, Mike Linacre, Mark Wilson, Carol Myford, Mary Garner, and Jennifer Randall. Students in my seminars at Emory University on Rasch Measurement Theory, Researcher-Constructed Measures, and Theories of Measurement in the Social and Behavioral Sciences helped me to improve the conceptualization and presentation of my ideas regarding invariant measurement. During the last stages of preparing the manuscript for publication, Aminah Perkins provided invaluable assistance in addressing numerous last minute substantive and organizational challenges. I would also like to thank the reviewers of the manuscript: Ralph De-Ayala (University of Nebraska – Lincoln), Ric Luecht (University of North Carolina – Greensboro), Carol Myford (University of Illinois at Chicago), and Jennifer Randall (University of Massachusetts, Amherst). I would also like to thank Debra Riegert of Routledge who served as a supportive editor throughout the preparation of the manuscript.

About the Author

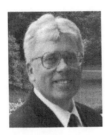

Dr. George Engelhard, Jr. is a professor of educational measurement and policy in the Division of Educational Studies at Emory University. Professor Engelhard received his Ph.D. from The University of Chicago in the MESA (measurement, evaluation, and statistical analysis) program. Professor Engelhard is co-editor of four books, and the author or co-author of over 125 journal articles, book chapters, and monographs. He serves on national technical advisory committees on educational measurement and policy for several states including Georgia, Louisiana, Michigan, New Jersey, Ohio, Pennsylvania, and Washington. He is a past president of the Georgia Educational Research Association. Professor Engelhard has received numerous awards and fellowships including a National Academy of Education/Spencer Foundation Fellowship Award, a Lilly Post-Doctoral Teaching Award, and a Writing Across the Curriculum Project Award. He is a fellow of the American Educational Research Association.

Part I

Introduction

Introduction and Overview

Rasch (1960) has devised a truly new approach to psychometric problems ... [that yields] non-arbitrary measures.

(Loevinger, 1965, p. 151)

[in the Rasch model] subjects θ [location on the latent variable] may be estimated "item-selection free", i.e., independently of the items sampled or selected for their measurement, and item δ's [item difficulties] may be determined "population free," i.e. independently of the particular subjects sampled or selected for measurement.

(Mokken, 1971, p. 110)

This chapter provides an introduction to issues related to invariant measurement in the social, behavioral, and health sciences. Invariant measurement has its genesis in the work of numerous measurement theorists during the 20th century. One of the clearest statements of invariant measurement is found in the work of Georg Rasch (1960/1980, 1977).

Rasch was a Danish mathematician who developed a new philosophical perspective on measurement based on his concept of "specific objectivity" and invariant comparisons between items and persons.[1] His ideas were originally presented in highly technical forms that were not easily accessible to many research workers in the human sciences. An example of Rasch's technical writing is given below:

The specifically objective comparison of two objects O_λ and O_ν and two agents A_i and A_j is based on the respective differences

---

1 Researchers who are interested in a biographical description of Georg Rasch's life should consult a dissertation written by Lina Wøhlk Olsen at the University of Copenhagen (http://www.rasch.org/olsen.htm). Another good source of biographical information on Rasch is the Foreword to Rasch's book (1960/1980) by Ben Wright.

(VI:8) $\xi'_{\lambda i} - \xi'_{vi} = \omega'_{\lambda} - \omega'_{v}$

and

(VI:9) $\xi'_{vi} - \xi'_{vj} = \alpha'_{i} - \alpha'_{j},$

the right hand expression of which are denoted: the elementary comparators.

If this condition is satisfied the frame of reference is called *latently additive*, while the comparisons between objects or between agents are called *latently subtractive*.

In passing one may observe the comparisons by means of the elementary comparators constitute interval measurements of the ω'- and α'-scales. A closer analysis of the relationship, thus hinted at, between the two concepts: measurement and comparison seems called for. (Rasch, 1977, p. 80)

The last line of this quote, "A closer analysis of the relationship thus hinted at, between the two concepts: measurement and comparison seems called for …" (Rasch, 1977, p. 80) becomes the basis for conceptualizing invariant measurement from the perspective of comparisons between items and persons. The concept of objective and invariant comparisons is an important theme in Rasch measurement specifically, and in invariant measurement more generally. One of the key developers and proponents of Rasch measurement was Professor Benjamin D. Wright at the University of Chicago.[2] Wright took the original work of Rasch and worked out the details of translating Rasch measurement models into useful and practical approaches to measurement in the social, behavioral, and health sciences.

The first section of this chapter describes the idea of variable maps. Next, a section describing logits (log-odd units) is included. The third section introduces the five requirements of invariant measurement. This is followed by a section that provides a description of the dichotomous Rasch model that includes an introduction to item and person response functions. The fifth section introduces Ben Wright's views on the method and meaning of Rasch

---

2   Professor Benjamin D. Wright of the University of Chicago first encountered Georg Rasch's revolutionary ideas about measurement during the 1960s while Rasch was a visiting professor at Chicago. Ben Wright went on to develop many enhancements and extensions to Rasch's measurement models in collaboration with numerous students and colleagues. Most of the developments described in this book can be traced either directly or indirectly to the work of Ben Wright. I was a graduate student and colleague of Ben Wright, and this book is strongly influenced by Ben's contributions to the advancement of the principles of Rasch measurement theory.

measurement based on a one-page summary that he created in the early 1980s. Next, an illustrative data set that addresses the measurement of the quality of home environments of preschool children is described. Finally, a summary and discussion of the key points in this chapter are highlighted.

Variable Maps

Variable maps provide an organizing concept for viewing the measurement process. A variable map provides a visual display of the underlying latent variable in a format similar to our ideal vision of a measuring instrument. The major goal of invariant measurement is to create a variable map with the simultaneous location of both item and persons on a line that represents the construct being measured. For example, yardsticks and thermometers provide familiar examples of what most people think of as measuring instruments. It is also possible in the social, behavioral, and health sciences to develop "yardsticks" that can be used to represent the important latent variables and constructs that researchers use to represent key ideas regarding how the world works.

Figure 1.1 provides a prototypical variable map. First, the researcher identifies the intended latent variable or construct that the scale is designed to measure. In essence, the variable map provides a visual display that answers the following question: What is the latent variable (construct)? Column 1 provides units for the measuring instrument on a logit scale. In the first stage of the process, the logit scale can simply be viewed as being metaphorically comparable to the inches or centimeters that define our units of measurement on a yardstick. The logit scale is described later in this chapter. Column 2 provides the first step in the process of developing an operational definition of our latent variable. The researcher must develop a conception, definition, and description of the characteristics of persons who have low, moderate, and high levels on the latent variable. For example, if the construct is mathematics achievement, then the researcher begins by defining this latent variable in terms of a vision of what students need to know and be able to do at different levels on the latent variable of mathematics achievement. Column 3 represents the next step in the construction of a scale. Particular items are created to represent a framework for collecting observations that will inform us regarding inferences of where persons are located on the latent variable. To continue the example using mathematics achievement as the latent variable, it is necessary to construct items that reflect low levels of mathematics achievement (e.g., single-digit addition) through items with midrange levels of difficulty (e.g., double-digit addition) to items with high levels of difficulty (e.g., division of fractions). The researcher also decides on the response format that will be used to collect ratings. There are a variety of formats that can be used including simple dichotomous ratings (0 = not present, 1 = present), or in the case of mathematics achievement the researcher might score multiple-choice items

Logit Scale	Persons	Items
	What is the latent variable (construct)?	
5.00		*[Hard items]*
4.00	High values on the latent variable	
3.00		
2.00		
1.00		
.00	Midrange values on the latent variable	*[Moderately difficult items]*
-1.00		
-2.00		
-3.00		
-4.00	Low values on the latent variable	
-5.00		*[Easy Items]*

What is the response format or rating scale used?
- Dichotomous (x=0, 1)
- Polytomous (x=0, 1, 2, 3 ...)

Figure 1.1   Prototypical Variable Map.

as incorrect (x = 0) or correct (x = 1). It should be stressed at this point in the measurement process that the description of persons and items are hypothesized to have particular locations on the latent variable. In later stages of the measurement process, these operational definitions will be empirically examined and the hypothesized locations evaluated with data. The overarching goal of measurement is to locate both persons and items simultaneously on the latent variable that can be visually displayed as a variable map. Rasch measurement models provide the psychometric theory for accomplishing this task of variable map construction.

Figure 1.2 presents an example of a hypothesized variable map. The underlying construct represents levels of learning stimulation available in a person's home environment based on Monsaas and Engelhard (1996). Column 1 is the logit scale. Column 2 provides brief descriptions of the home environments of preschool children who have three levels of stimulation: low, midrange, and high levels of learning stimulation. The last column provides sample items that are hypothesized to represent different levels of difficulty. These items range from objects that are relatively easy to find in most homes with preschool children (toys to teach colors and shapes) to objects that are harder to find (family subscribes to a magazine).

Variable maps are conceptually similar to yardsticks, thermometers, clocks and other measuring instruments that provide visual representations of latent variables, such as height, temperature and time. In essence, a variable map is a visual version of the operational definition of the latent variable or construct that include a scale, person descriptions, and illustrative items. There are numerous examples of early versions of variable maps that include

---

What is the latent variable?

The latent variable is the learning stimulation available in the home environments of preschool children.

Logit Scale	Home Environments of Preschool Children	Home Observations [items]
5.00		[Hard items]
4.00	Home environment provides enriching and stimulating learning opportunities [High learning stimulation]	Family subscribes to a magazine
3.00		Family buys and reads a daily newspaper
2.00		
1.00	Home environment provides some enriching and stimulating learning opportunities [Midrange learning stimulation]	Ten books visible
.00		Ten children's books visible
-1.00		[Moderately difficult items]
-2.00		
-3.00	Home environment provides few enriching and stimulating learning opportunities [Low learning stimulation]	Toys to teach numbers
-4.00		Toys to teach colors and shapes
-5.00		[Easy items]

What is the response format or rating scale used?

Dichotomous scores are used with not present coded as zero (x=0), and present coded as one (x=1)

Figure 1.2 Example of hypothesized variable map for a Learning Stimulation Scale (Home Environment).

a scale representing ability in reading by Thorndike (1914), English composition (Thorndike, 1916), the scaling of the Binet Test Questions for measuring intelligence (Thurstone, 1925), and the measurement of attitudes (Thurstone & Chave, 1929). Recent examples of variable maps include the Lexile Framework for Reading, and the Quantile Framework for Mathematics. The Lexile variable map can be found at the following website: http://www.lexile.com/m/uploads/maps/Lexile-Map.pdf, while the Quantile Framework can be found at: http://quantiles.com/pdf/Quantile%20Map.pdf. Stone, Wright, and Stenner (1999) trace the historical origins of mapping, as well as a description of how variable maps can be used to conceptualize, develop, calibrate, monitor, and revise our measures. Variable maps are useful displays that can be presented in a variety of formats that all convey the key idea of an underlying line that represents the location of items and persons on a latent variable or construct. As is the case with geographical maps, it is recognized that we are presenting a simplified representation of a complex and multidimensional construct in two-dimensions (Monmonmier, 1996). Further details regarding the steps necessary to construct variable maps are presented in Chapter 4.

What Are Logits?

In order to understand the Rasch model, it is important to have a sense of the underlying units used in the logit scale. Essentially, logits provide the units used to locate the marks on our measuring instruments. In the same sense that rulers are divided into units based on inches or centimeters, the logit defines the units underlying the Rasch model. The word logit is short for the phrase "log-odds unit." Logits are a non-linear transformation of proportions used to create a linear scale that is more likely to have equal units (Ashton, 1972). In biometrics, similar units based on the normal curve are called normits (Bock & Jones, 1968). Other nonlinear transformations of proportions include probits (Finney, 1952), and an arc-sine function that has been proposed by Bock and Jones (1968). These transformations share the desirable property that a non-linear transformation is used to create linear scales that are more likely to have equal units than the original proportions. In essence, the purpose of the logit transformation is to provide a non-linear transformation of proportion scores for items and persons that provide values that are more likely to have equal units.

The logistic transformation of proportions produces values that can range from $-\infty$ to $+\infty$ with most logit values found in practice falling between -5.00 and 5.00. The logistic transformation is defined as follows:

$$\textbf{Logit} = \Psi[x] = ln[x/1 - x] \qquad [1]$$

where the symbol, $\Psi[\chi]$, is the symbolic representation of the logistic transformation for x, and ln represents the symbol for the natural logarithm.

Person logits can be defined by substituting proportion correct, p, defined as number of correct items/total number of items for x in Equation 1. This is shown in Equation 2.

$$\textbf{Person Logit} = \Psi[p] = ln[\,p\,/(1-p)] \qquad [2]$$

Item logits can be defined in a similar fashion by substituting 1 minus the item *p-values* for x in Equation 1. For items, the *p-value* is defined as the number of correct responses divided by total number of persons who responded to the item. This is shown in Equation 3.

$$\textbf{Item Logit} = \Psi[\text{p-value}] = ln[\text{p-value}/(1-\text{p-value})] \qquad [3]$$

Conversely, it is possible to move from logits to proportion correct or *p-values* as follows:

$$\textbf{Proportion} = \exp(\text{logit})/\,[1 + \exp(\text{logit})] \qquad [4]$$

where exp(x) represents e^x and e $\approx$ 2.71828 ... Table 1.1 presents values that illustrate the relationship between proportions and logits for both items and persons. Column 1 lists the logit scale from –5.00 to 5.00. As pointed out earlier, this scale actually can range from $-\infty$ to $+\infty$, although most values fall within the range shown in Table 1.1. Column 1 shows how item difficulty is defined on the logit scale with hard items having positive values and easy items having negative values. The entries in Column 2 can be viewed as the customary item *p-values*, while the entries in Column 3 present the proportion-correct scores for persons. It should be noted the logit scale for item difficulty goes in the opposite direction from the *p-values*. In other words, a *p-value* of .88 (Logit = –2.00) would be considered a very easy item, while an item with a *p-value* of .12 (Logit = 2.00) is a hard item.

According to Wright (1993), these logit measures for items and persons have a number of desirable characteristics:

> [w]hen any pair of logit measurements have been made with respect to the same origin on the same scale, the difference between them is obtained merely by subtraction and is also in Logits ... the logit scale is unaffected by variations in the distribution of measures that have been previously made, or by which items ... may have been used to construct and calibrate the scale. The logit scale can be made entirely independent of the particular group of items that happen to be included in a test this time, or the particular samplings of persons that happen to have been used to calibrate these items. (p. 288)

Logits in Rasch measurement theory can be also defined as follows:

$$\text{Logit} = Ln\left(\frac{P_{i1}}{P_{i0}}\right) = \theta - \delta_i \qquad [5]$$

where P_{i1} is the conditional probability of scoring 1 on item i, P_{i0} is the conditional probability of scoring 0 on item i, and θ is the location of the person on the latent variable. The term P_{i1} / P_{i0} (Probability of Success)/ (Probability of Failure) represents the odds of success. The log (*Ln*) of this term is called

Table 1.1   Logit Scale

Logit Scale	Items: ln [(1-p)/p]	Persons: ln [p/(1-p)]
	Proportion-correct for items, p-values	Proportion-correct score for persons
	Hard item	High achieving persons
5.00	0.01	0.99
4.50	0.01	0.99
4.00	0.02	0.98
3.50	0.03	0.97
3.00	0.05	0.95
2.50	0.08	0.92
2.00	0.12	0.88
1.50	0.18	0.82
1.00	0.27	0.73
0.50	0.38	0.62
0.00	0.50	0.50
-0.50	0.62	0.38
-1.00	0.73	0.27
-1.50	0.82	0.18
-2.00	0.88	0.12
-2.50	0.92	0.08
-3.00	0.95	0.05
-3.50	0.97	0.03
-4.00	0.98	0.02
-4.50	0.99	0.01
-5.00	0.99	0.01
	Easy item	Low achieving person

Note. Proportions correct for items (*p-value*) represent item difficulties. In a parallel fashion, proportion-correct scores for persons are defined as the number of correct items divided by total number of items for a person.

log-odds. This transformation produces log-odds units called logits. It should be noted that the logits are simply defined as a comparison or difference between the location of a person on the latent variable and item difficulty. This simple structure is essential in the realization of invariant measurement. It also highlights Rasch's observation that comparisons (in this case, between person and item locations on the latent variable) can form the basis for useful measurement models.

As with other aspects of invariant measurement, whether or not an equal interval logit scale is achieved with a particular set of data depends on how well the data fit the model and the underlying theory of Rasch measurement. If the model-data fit is good, then equal interval scales can be approximated. Future chapters provide more detail and a discussion of model-data fit.

There are a number of different perspectives that can be used to justify the logistic transformation of proportions or *p-values* to logits. First, it has been shown that the logistic distribution provides a good approximation to the normal distribution after division by a constant (1.7). Second, the logistic transformation is a member of the family of exponential distributions that have been shown to have many desirable statistical properties (Barndorf-Nielson, 1978). It can also be viewed as representing random within-person variation related to underlying or latent response processes. Finally, logits can be simply viewed as one of several possible transformations of proportions to create a linear scale.

The Dichotomous Rasch Model

Figure 1.3 summarizes the form of person response functions for the dichotomous Rasch model. The upper panel represents the responses, x_{A1}, of a single person (Person A) to a set of items with a dichotomous response (e.g., 1 = correct response, and 0 = incorrect response). The equation for the dichotomous Rasch model with the probability of a correct response expressed as a function of the logits is shown. The logits for a person response function are defined as the differences between a person's location on the latent variable, θ_A, and the difficulties of a set of items, δ_i. This equation is shown graphically as a monotonically decreasing logistic curve.

The lower panel in Figure 1.3 gives the equation for the dichotomous Rasch model with the probability of an *incorrect* response expressed as a person response function related to the logits. As before, the person response function for incorrect responses is defined as the differences between a person's location on the latent variable, θ_A, and the difficulties of a set of items, δ_i. This equation is also presented graphically.

In a parallel fashion, Figure 1.4 summarizes the form of item response functions for the dichotomous Rasch model. The top panel represents the responses, x_{n1}, of person n to a single item (Item 1) with a dichotomous response (e.g., 1 = correct response, and 0 = incorrect response). The equation

Probability of a correct response ($x_{Ai} = 1$)

$$Pr(x_{Ai} = 1|\theta_A, \delta_i) = \exp(\theta_A - \delta_i)/\ [1 + \exp(\theta_A - \delta_i)]$$

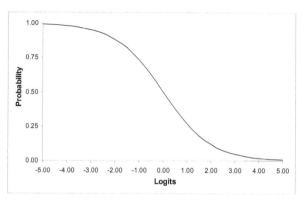

Probability of an incorrect response ($x_{Ai} = 0$)

$$Pr(x_A = 0|\ \theta_A, \delta_i) = 1\ /\ [1 + \exp(\theta_A - \delta_i)]$$

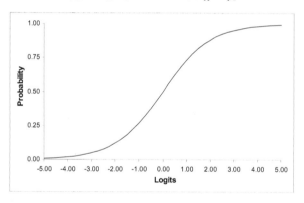

Figure 1.3 Person response functions for the dichotomous Rasch model: Person A ($\theta A = .00$).

for the dichotomous Rasch model with the probability of a correct response expressed as a function of the logits is also presented. The logits for an item response function are defined as the differences between person's locations on the latent variable, θ_n, and the difficulty of Item 1, δ_1. This equation is also shown graphically in Figure 1.4.

The bottom half of Figure 1.4 gives the equation for the dichotomous Rasch model with the probability of an *incorrect* response expressed as a function of the logits. As before, the item response function for incorrect responses is defined as the differences between person's locations on the latent variable, θ_n, and the difficulty of Item 1, δ_1.

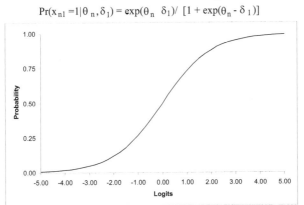

Probability of a correct response ($x_{nl} = 1$)

$$\Pr(x_{nl} = 1 | \theta_n, \delta_1) = \exp(\theta_n \; \delta_1) / \; [1 + \exp(\theta_n - \delta_1)]$$

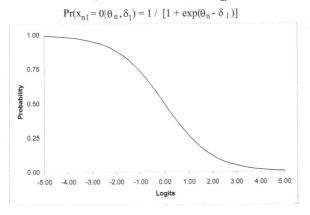

Probability of an incorrect response ($x_{nl} = 0$)

$$\Pr(x_{nl} = 0 | \theta_n, \delta_1) = 1 / \; [1 + \exp(\theta_n - \delta_1)]$$

Figure 1.4 Item Response Functions for the dichotomous Rasch model: Item 1 ($\delta 1 = .00$).

Figures 1.3 and 1.4 highlight the duality between item and person response functions. These concepts are utilized throughout this book to explore issues related to invariant measurement.

Five Requirements of Invariant Measurement

The goal of measurement is to develop variable maps that can be used to represent the locations of both persons and items on a latent variable of substantive and theoretical interest. In order to develop useful scales for measurement, there are five essential requirements of invariant measurement. These requirements are briefly presented in Figure 1.5. These five requirements are

---

Five Requirements for Invariant Measurement

Person measurement:

1. The measurement of persons must be independent of the particular items that happen to be used for the measuring: *Item-invariant measurement of persons.*

2. A more able person must always have a better chance of success on an item than a less able person: *non-crossing person response functions.*

Item calibration:

3. The calibration of the items must be independent of the particular persons used for calibration: *Person-invariant calibration of test items.*

4. Any person must have a better chance of success on an easy item than on a more difficult item: *non-crossing item response functions.*

Variable map:

5. Items and person must be simultaneously located on a single underlying latent variable: *variable map.*

Figure 1.5

based on the philosophical and theoretical framework of Rasch measurement models. This list is presented as a set of requirements rather than assumptions because scales and instruments must meet or approximate these conditions in order to yield useful inferences that generalize beyond the particular group of persons used to calibrate the items, as well as generalize beyond the particular items or observations used to measure the persons. These requirements reflect an ideal-type model for measurement in the human sciences.

The first two requirements are related to person measurement. First of all, invariant measurement requires that a person's location on the latent variable should not be dependent on particular items used to determine the location. This suggests that calibrated items with known locations on the latent variable can be used in an exchangeable manner. Item-invariant measurement is essential. The second requirement related to person measurement states that a more able person must always have a better chance of success on an item than a less able person. It has not been widely recognized that crossing person response curves can play havoc with the meaning and invariance of measurement scales across persons. The substantive impact of crossing person response functions is presented in Figure 1.6.

Panels A and C illustrate item invariant measurement with the ordering of the three persons being the same over item subsets: A < B < C. Panels B

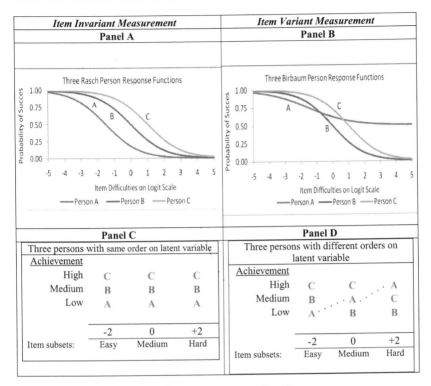

Figure 1.6   The impact of crossing person response functions.

and D illustrate item variant measurement with persons ordered differently depending on the item subsets. For easy items, order of the persons is A < B < C, while for the hard items B < C < A. Person A has moved from having the lowest achievement on the easy items to having the highest achievement on the hard items. It is clear that these three persons are not being measured on the same latent variable when the person response functions cross. Crossing person response functions are described in Perkins and Engelhard (2009), and Lumsden (1977) provides a very nice description of the consequences of ignoring the concept of person response functions.

Requirements 3 and 4 address issues related to item calibration. Item locations on the latent variable should be independent of the particular persons or subsets of persons used to calibrate the items. This requirement is called person-invariant calibration of items. Studies of differential item functioning (DIF) and measurement invariance are conducted to determine whether or not item locations are invariant across various subgroups. If the item locations are not invariant across groups, then this may be evidence of various sorts of item bias. Item response functions that cross make it impossible to locate items on the latent variable that are invariant over subgroups. This interaction effect has the substantive implication that items above the point where the curves cross have one difficulty order, while items below the crossing point of two item response functions have a different difficulty order for persons in this segment of the logit scale. This is illustrated in Figure 1.7 (Wright, 1997).

Panel A provides the item response functions for five vocabulary items that fit the Rasch model. It is clear that the ordering of the items by difficulty for three subgroups of persons on the ability or logit scale is invariant over the 1st, 2nd, and 3rd subgroups. Panel C shows how the items are located on the variable map for these three subgroups of persons. Evidence for person-invariant

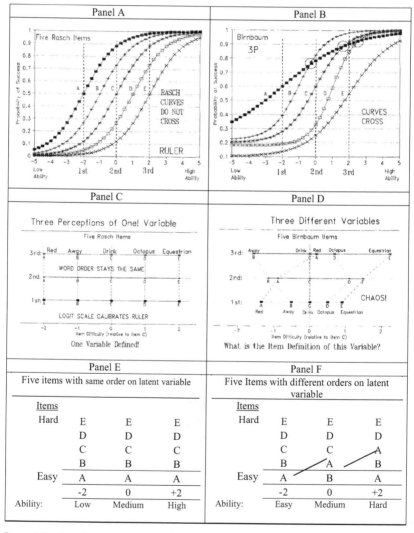

Figure 1.7   The impact of crossing item response functions on the location of items on the latent variable.

measurement is illustrated by Panels A and C. Panel B presents the item response functions for another item response model (Birnbaum, 1968) that adds parameters that permit the item response functions to cross. In this case, the ordering of the item difficulties is not invariant over the three groups of persons. The differential mapping of the vocabulary items onto the underlying latent variable is show in Panel D for five Birnbaum items. Panels E illustrates invariance, while Panel F illustrates how item orders are not invariant over the three subgroups of persons that range from low to high ability. For example in Panel E, if item response functions do not cross, then item order from easy to hard remains the same: A < B < C < D < E. When item response functions are allowed to cross, then item order is not invariant over subgroups of persons as shown in Panel F: A < B < C for the low ability group, while item order from easy to hard is B < C < A.

The fifth requirement of unidimensionality is fundamental for invariant measurement. Our instruments must be designed to represent and measure one latent variable at a time. In the physical sciences, we do not attempt to measure height and weight with the same instrument even though there is clearly a relationship between these two variables.

Invariant measurement embodies many of the theoretical advances implicit in modern measurement theory. Rasch measurement models reflect what have been called the new rules of measurement that can serve as a guide to measurement practices in the 21st century (Embretson, 1996). The requirements of invariant measurement are further developed in Chapter 2, and they are elaborated on throughout this book.

Method and Meaning of Rasch Measurement

In 1989, Ben Wright constructed a one-page summary of Rasch measurement that is shown in Figure 1.8. This summary highlights the essential features of the dichotomous Rasch model.

This summary also highlights the elegance of a simple, but powerful, model that can be used to meet the five requirements of invariant measurement described in the previous section. Figure 1.8 may need some updating, but the framework remains remarkably sound for introducing the method and meaning of measurement. For now, the key parts of Figure 1.8 are the two boxes labeled Rasch Measurement. The "Data" box indicates the essential structure of the observations that form the empirical basis for measurement. This illustration highlights the idea that persons ($n = 1$ to N) respond to a set of items ($i = 1$ to L) with dichotomous responses ($X_{ni} = 0,1$). The "Measurement Model" box presents the equation for the dichotomous Rasch model that can be used to model data. P_{ni} represents the probability of person n responding to item i with a response (X_{ni}) of zero or one. The Rasch model is presented in both exponential and log-odds form. In future chapters, Figure 1.8 serves as a

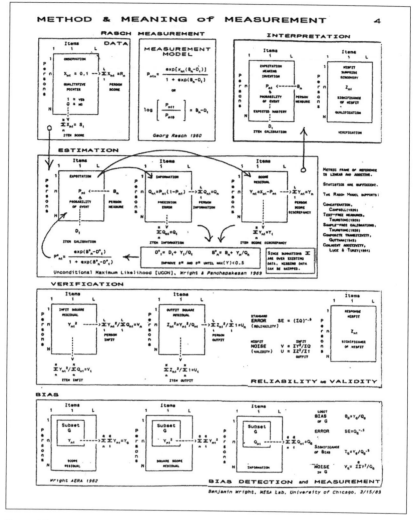

Figure 1.8   One page summary of the dichotomous Rasch model (Classroom handout, 1989).

guide for addressing issues of estimation, interpretation, verification and bias. The other panels in Figure 1.8 are elaborated on in later chapters.

Illustrative Data Set: Measuring the Home Environment

This section provides a brief introduction to a Rasch analysis of an illustrative data set developed to measure selected aspects of the home environment. The variable map in Figure 1.9 is based on data collected as part of a study conducted by Monsaas and Engelhard (1996). The purpose of this study was

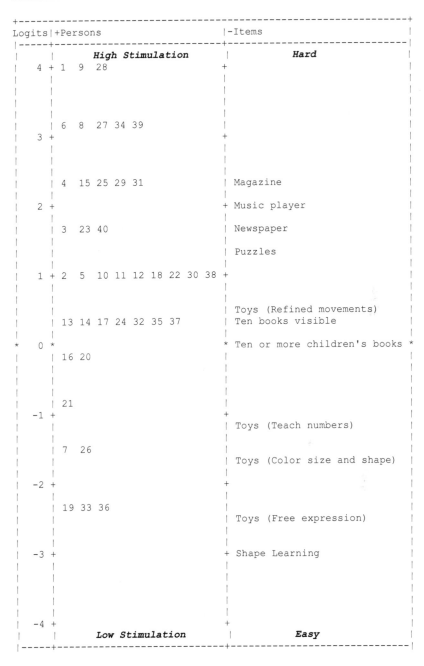

```
+--------------------------------------------------------------+
Logits|+Persons                      |-Items                   |
|-----+-----------------------------+-------------------------|
|     |          High Stimulation   |         Hard            |
|  4 + 1   9   28                    +                         |
|     |                             |                         |
|     |                             |                         |
|     |                             |                         |
|     | 6   8   27 34 39            |                         |
|  3 +                              +                         |
|     |                             |                         |
|     |                             |                         |
|     |                             |                         |
|     | 4   15 25 29 31             | Magazine                |
|     |                             |                         |
|  2 +                              + Music player            |
|     |                             |                         |
|     | 3   23 40                   | Newspaper               |
|     |                             |                         |
|     |                             | Puzzles                 |
|     |                             |                         |
|  1 + 2   5   10 11 12 18 22 30 38 +                         |
|     |                             |                         |
|     |                             |                         |
|     |                             | Toys (Refined movements)|
|     | 13 14 17 24 32 35 37        | Ten books visible       |
|     |                             |                         |
*  0 *                              * Ten or more children's books *
|     | 16 20                       |                         |
|     |                             |                         |
|     |                             |                         |
|     |                             |                         |
|     | 21                          |                         |
| -1 +                              +                         |
|     |                             | Toys (Teach numbers)    |
|     |                             |                         |
|     | 7   26                      |                         |
|     |                             | Toys (Color size and shape)|
|     |                             |                         |
| -2 +                              +                         |
|     |                             |                         |
|     | 19 33 36                    |                         |
|     |                             | Toys (Free expression)  |
|     |                             |                         |
|     |                             |                         |
| -3 +                              + Shape Learning          |
|     |                             |                         |
|     |                             |                         |
|     |                             |                         |
|     |                             |                         |
| -4 +                              +                         |
|     |          Low Stimulation    |         Easy            |
|-----+-----------------------------+-------------------------|
```

Figure 1.9   Empirical Variable Map for Home Environment (Learning Stimulation).

to examine changes in home environments based on an early intervention program called Preschool Parent Partners. This section presents data based on one of the subscales of the Home Observation for Measurement of the Environment (HOME) instrument developed by Caldwell and Bradley (1984). The subscale selected was designed to measure the level of learning stimulation in the home environments for pre-school children. This Learning Stimulation Scale is composed of 11 items, and these are described in Table 1.2.

A review of the HOME instrument is provided by Boehm (1985). A revised version of the HOME instrument is described in Toksika and Sylva (2004).

Table 1.3 provides the responses for the 11-item Learning Stimulation Scale collected from the home environments of 40 preschool children. The entries in Table 1.3 represent teacher observations based on home visits regarding the absence (x = 0) or presence (x = 1) of various objects in the home environments of these 40 preschool children. Table 1.3 illustrates the basic form of the data that are analyzed in the social, behavioral, and health sciences. This form of data includes tables with rows representing persons and columns representing items with the responses of person to items (x = 0, 1) as entries in the cells of the table with 0 = not present, and 1 = present.

Table 1.2   Learning Stimulation Scale

Item	Description of Item	Not Present (x = 0)	Present (x = 1)
1	Child has toys which teach color, size, and shape.	w	w
2	Child has three or more puzzles.	w	w
3	Child has record player and at least five children's records.	w	w
4	Child has toys permitting free expression	w	w
5	Child has toys or games requiring refined movements.	w	w
6	Child has toys or games which help teach numbers.	w	w
7	Child has at least 10 children's books.	w	w
8	At least 10 books are visible in the apartment.	w	w
9	Family buys and reads a daily newspaper.	w	w
10	Family subscribes to at least one magazine.	w	w
11	Child is encouraged to learn shapes.	w	w

Adapted from Caldwell, B.M. & Bradley, R.H. Home observation for measurement of environment. University of Arkansas, 1984.

Table 1.3   Observed Ratings for the Home Environments of 40 Children on the Learning Stimulation Scale

Child	Items										
	1	*2*	*3*	*4*	*5*	*6*	*7*	*8*	*9*	*10*	*11*
1	1	1	1	1	1	1	1	1	1	1	1
2	1	0	0	1	0	1	1	1	1	0	1
3	1	1	0	1	1	1	1	1	0	0	1
4	1	0	1	1	1	1	1	1	0	1	1
5	1	0	1	1	1	0	1	0	0	1	1
6	1	1	0	1	1	1	1	1	1	1	1
7	1	1	0	1	0	0	0	0	0	0	0
8	1	1	1	1	1	1	1	0	1	1	1
9	1	1	1	1	1	1	1	1	1	1	1
10	1	0	0	1	1	1	0	1	1	0	1
11	1	1	0	1	0	1	1	1	0	0	1
12	1	0	0	1	1	1	1	1	0	0	1
13	1	0	1	1	0	1	0	1	0	0	1
14	1	0	1	1	0	1	0	1	0	0	1
15	1	1	1	1	1	1	1	1	0	0	1
16	1	0	0	1	0	1	0	0	1	0	1
17	1	0	0	1	1	1	1	0	0	0	1
18	1	1	0	1	0	1	1	0	1	0	1
19	0	0	0	0	0	1	0	0	0	0	1
20	1	0	0	1	0	1	0	1	0	0	1
21	1	0	0	1	1	0	0	0	0	0	1
22	0	0	1	1	0	1	1	1	1	0	1
23	1	0	1	1	1	0	1	1	0	1	1
24	0	0	1	1	1	0	0	1	1	0	1
25	1	1	0	1	1	1	1	1	0	1	1
26	0	0	0	0	0	0	1	0	1	0	1
27	1	1	1	1	1	1	1	1	0	1	1
28	1	1	1	1	1	1	1	1	1	1	1
29	1	1	1	1	1	1	1	1	0	0	1
30	1	1	0	1	0	1	1	0	1	0	1
31	1	1	0	1	1	1	1	1	1	0	1
32	1	0	0	1	1	1	1	0	0	0	1

(continued)

Table 1.3   Continued

| | | | | | Items | | | | | |
Child	1	2	3	4	5	6	7	8	9	10	11
33	0	0	0	1	0	0	0	0	0	0	1
34	1	1	0	1	1	1	1	1	1	1	1
35	1	0	0	1	0	1	0	1	0	1	1
36	1	0	0	0	0	1	0	0	0	0	0
37	1	1	0	1	1	1	0	0	0	0	1
38	1	0	0	1	1	1	1	0	0	1	1
39	1	1	1	1	1	1	1	1	1	0	1
40	1	1	0	1	0	1	1	1	1	0	1

Note: Cell entries indicate that the items are present (x = 1) or not present (x = 0) for the home environments of 40 children.

Discussion and Summary

The major aim of this book is to make Rasch models and the concept of invariant measurement accessible to a wider audience. It is designed to provide sufficient detail to allow researchers to gain some insight into the underlying philosophy and guiding principles of sound measurement based on the concept of invariance. Future research in the social, behavioral, and health sciences depends in a fundamental way on the development of psychometrically defensible instruments that measure the key constructs that comprise the substantive theories in these fields. The intent of this book is to play at least a small role towards helping researchers achieve this goal.

A main theme of this chapter emphasizes the idea of variable maps, and the key importance of variable maps for measurement in the social, behavioral, and health sciences. There are five requirements of invariant measurement that are necessary for developing useful variable maps to adequately develop and represent measures of latent variables and constructs. Rasch measurement theory provides a framework for viewing the methods and meaning of measurement that under appropriate conditions can yield invariant measurement. A non-linear transformation based on logits (log-odd units) provides the underlying mechanism for the first step in developing useful units for our scales. The dichotomous Rasch model includes both item and person response functions that can be used to build variable maps with both person and item locations mapped onto the same latent variable.

It is appropriate to end this chapter with an extensive quote by E.L. Thorndike (see Figure 1.10) who was a key measurement theorist more than a century ago: It is hoped that this book uncovers some of the "mysteries of the specialist" in regards to invariant measurement for all researchers who are committed to creating psychometrically sound scales and instruments in the social, behavioral, and health sciences.

CHAPTER I.

INTRODUCTION.

Mathematics and Measurements.

THE power to follow abstract mathematical arguments is rare and its development in the course of school education is rarer still. For example, few of us are able to understand the symbols or processes used in the quotation on the following page. Yet it is a rather easy sample of the discussions from which the student is expected to gain insight into the theory of measurement appropriate to the variable phenomena with which the mental sciences have to deal.

It would be unfortunate if the ability to understand and use the newer methods of measurement were dependent upon the mathematical capacity and training which were required to derive and formulate them. The great majority of thinkers would then be deprived of the most efficient weapon in investigations of mental and social facts, and adequate statistical studies could be made only by the few students of psychology, sociology, economics and education who happened to be also proficient mathematicians.

There is, happily, nothing in the general principles of modern statistical theory but refined common sense, and little in the technique resulting from them that general intelligence can not readily master. A new method devised by a mathematician is likely to be expressed by him in terms intelligible only to those with mathematical training, and to be explained by him through an abstract derivation which only those with mathematical training and capacity can understand. It may, nevertheless, be possible to explain its meaning and use in common language to a common-sense thinker. With time what were the mysteries of the specialist become the property of all. To aid this process in the case of certain recent contributions to statistical theory is one of the leading aims of this book. Knowledge will be presupposed of only the elements of arithmetic and algebra. Artificial symbols will be used only when they are really convenient. Concrete illustrations will always accompany and often replace abstract laws.

1   1

Thorndike, E.L. An Introduction to the Theory of Mental and Social Measurements. Teachers College, Columbia University, 1904. (p. 1)

Figure 1.10 Thorndike Quote on Mathematics and Measurement.

Part II

Conceptual and Theoretical Issues

Chapter 2

Invariant Measurement

Einstein, however, was not truly a relativist ... beneath all of his theories, including relativity, was a quest for invariants ... and the goal of science was to discover it.

(Isaacson, 2007, p. 3)

Einstein briefly considered calling his creation Invariance Theory.

(Isaacson, 2007, p. 132)

I first encountered the idea of invariant measurement in an article by Ben Wright (1968). His work was originally presented at the 1967 Invitational Conference on Testing Problems hosted by Educational Testing Service in New York City. Wright described the limitations of current approaches to measurement, and he very succinctly stated an ideal view of invariant measurement in the social sciences:

> First, the calibration of measuring instruments must be independent of those objects that happen to be used for the calibration. Second, the measurement of objects must be independent of the instrument that happens to be used for the measuring. In practice, these conditions can only be approximated. But their approximation is what makes measurement objective. (p. 87)

Wright contrasted this view of what he called "objective measurement" with current practices in the social and behavioral sciences that yielded sample-dependent item calibrations, and person measurements that depended on the items included in a particular instrument. Wright pointed out that score meaning typically depends "not only on which items I took, but on who I was and the company I kept" (p. 85).

Rasch developed a set of requirements for measurement that he called "specific objectivity." These requirements form the seminal ideas for invariant measurement as described in this book. Specific objectivity informs the essential aspects of invariant measurement. Invariant measurement has a long history with numerous measurement theorists in addition to Rasch contributing to the quest for invariant measurement. A short history of measurement is described in Chapter 5, and Chapter 6 describes the quest for invariant measurement.

Problems related to invariant measurement played a key role in the development of the measurement theory of Rasch. As pointed out by Andrich (1988), Rasch presented "two principles of invariance for making comparisons that in an important sense precede, though inevitably lead to, measurement" (p. 18).

> [t]he comparison between two stimuli should be independent of which particular individuals were instrumental for the comparison; and it should also be independent of which stimuli within the considered class were or might also have been compared. Symmetrically, a comparison between two individuals should be independent of which particular stimuli within the class considered were instrumental for the comparison; and it should be independent of which other individuals were also compared, on the same or on some other occasion (Rasch, 1961, pp. 331–332).

It is clear in this quotation that Rasch recognized the importance of both sample-invariant item calibration (items viewed as stimuli) and item-invariant measurement of individuals.

The first section of this chapter provides a brief description of how measurement is defined in this book with the idea of variable maps featured as a key concept. Next, some of the philosophical issues underlying invariant measurement are presented. The following section describes the structure of measurement data, and introduces ideal-type measurement scales as conceptualized by Louis Guttman. The next section provides a description of the Rasch model for dichotomous data, and it develops a perspective on the Rasch model as a stochastic or probabilistic version of Guttman scaling that also includes an ideal-type perspective on measurement. Next, two simple examples of invariant measurement are provided to illustrate item-invariant person measurement and person-invariant item calibration. Finally, a summary of the key ideas in the chapter are highlighted and discussed.

What Is Measurement?

In this book, measurement in the social, behavioral, and health sciences is defined as the process of locating both persons and items on a line that represents a latent variable. The latent variable reflects the construct or attribute that the scale is designed to measure. This view of measurement reflects the idea that the responses of a person to a set of items are primarily a function of the location of the person (e.g., achievement level) and of the items (item difficulties) on the latent variable. This view of measurement is made visible by variable maps. Variable maps have also been called construct maps, item maps, curriculum maps, and Wright maps (in honor of Ben Wright). This view of measurement as the construction of a variable map echoes the ideal-type views of measurement in the physical sciences, as represented by instruments such as yardsticks to measure length, thermometers to measure temperature, and clocks to measure time.

A prototypical variable map was shown in Figure 1.1 in Chapter 1. In variable maps, the left column represents the underlying scale in log odd units (logits) that is to be constructed as a part of the measurement process. The second column indicates the location of persons on this latent variable with higher scores on the logit scale indicating more of the latent variable and lower values indicating less of the latent variable. The third column indicates the mapping of the items onto the same underlying latent variable with higher values indicating more difficult items, and lower values indicating easier items. The fourth column represents the responses that persons make to items on the scale with higher values or scores indicating that the responses are in a positive or increasing direction. As pointed out earlier, variable maps provide a useful visual representation and operational definition of the latent variable. For example, variable maps have become an integral part of the standard-setting process in a variety of assessment programs.

What Is Invariant Measurement?

Measurement can be defined as the assignment of numbers by rules to a set of persons or objects. The key to invariant measurement is to develop a set of rules and requirements that provide the opportunity to develop scales that possess a set of desirable properties. In order to accomplish this task, key measurement theorists, such as Louis Guttman and Georg Rasch, defined the requirements of their ideal-type scales. The five requirements of invariant measurement described in this book represent a key set of rules for defining ideal-type measurement. These rules are defined a priori, and they are not derived from any particular data set.

The concept of ideal-types is an important philosophical point that distinguishes Guttman scaling and Rasch models from other approaches to measurement based on statistical frameworks with a focus on fitting models to data. Guttman and Rasch models are based on measurement philosophies that place the models above the vagaries of imperfect data. In standard statistical approaches to data, the goal is to reproduce the observed data matrix as closely as possible, while the psychometric approach based on ideal-types is to create items and observations that hold the potential to meet the requirements of particular measurement models in order to realize the desirable properties of invariant measurement. The use of ideal-type models can be viewed as a fundamental and sound philosophical approach to the science of measurement in the human sciences.

In addition to the concept of ideal-types, it is important to keep in mind the duality between person measurement and item calibration (Mosier, 1940, 1941). The general functional relationship between the probability of a correct response and the logit scale is referred to here as an operating characteristic (OC) function with both person response functions and item response functions defined based on how the logits on the x-axis are operationalized. For example, an item response function is defined as an OC function for a single item with the x-axis defined as the differences between person locations and the location of the focus item. Conversely, a person response function is defined as an OC function for an individual person with the x-axis defined as the differences between the item locations (item difficulties) and location of the focus person.

Underlying the measurement philosophies of both Guttman and Rasch is the key idea that the requirements of our measurement models are falsifiable. In other words, we have to accept the possibility that our measures may not be working as intended for particular items sets and person groups. Falsifiability was a cornerstone of Karl Popper's view of science (1959, 1963), and when applied to measurement in the human sciences stresses that not all instruments or scales will meet the requirements of invariant measurement. Although Popper's views have been criticized as a general approach to science, the tenet of falsifiability has heuristic value within the context of developing scales that possess or approximate the ideal of invariant measurement.

Ideal-Type Scales and the Structure of Measurement Data

In order to explore the structure of measurement data that can yield invariant measurement, it is useful to imagine an ideal-type situation where the responses are simply a function of person and item locations on the latent variable. One of the clearest examples of this perspective is found in Louis Guttman's work on scaling. Guttman proposed a set of requirements for a perfect scale. Guttman Scaling is the technique he recommended for determining whether or not a set of items and person groups met the requirements of a perfect scale. Guttman determined these requirements based on an ideal-type perspective on scales. This approach is methodologically related to the concept of ideal types proposed by the German sociologist Max Weber. Coser (1977) described Weber's ideal type as follows:

> an ideal type is an analytical construct that serves the investigator as a measuring rod to ascertain similarities as well as deviations in concrete cases. It provides the basic method for comparative study ... Ideal types enable one to construct hypotheses linking them with the conditions that brought the phenomenon or event into prominence ... (pp. 223–224)

The concept of ideal types and the view of an ideal structure for measurement data places invariant measurement firmly within a strong methodological framework. As discussed earlier, this concept stresses the idea of falsifiability or refutability of requirements, and approaches issues of model-data fit from a particular perspective that sets it apart from other statistical approaches to data analyses. In particular, this ideal-type view of measurement focuses on the fitting of data to models. In other words, the model comes first with the requirements of good measurement, and the fit of the observed data to this ideal or theoretical model is the second step. The guiding variable map reflects the hypothesized structure of the latent variable defined by locations of items and persons, while the model-data fit provides a confirmation or disconfirmation of the variable map based on observed data. This can be contrasted with standard statistical practices that treat data as given with the major task of the researcher being to reproduce this data set as closely as possible with a tool kit of different statistical models.

A data matrix (persons by items) meets the requirements of a perfect Guttman scale when person scores reproduce the exact item responses in the data matrix.

> A particularly simple representation of the data would be to assign to each individual a numerical value and to each category of each attribute a numerical value such that, given the value of the individual and the values of the categories of an attribute, we could reproduce the observations of the individual on the attribute. (Guttman, 1944, p. 143)

Guttman sought a method for reproducing the item responses of each person based simply on a person's score (sum of correct answers).

Guttman proposed a variety of graphical and numerical methods for determining whether or not a "scale deviates from the ideal scale patterns" (Guttman, 1950, p. 77). Guttman's graphical method is called a scalogram. When persons and items are ordered and displayed in a table, then the data matrix form a distinctive triangular pattern for an ideal or perfect scale. This pattern is shown in the top section of Table 2.1 with index numbers 1 to 5. The person scores are listed in descending order (4 to 0) in column 2, and the items are ordered from easy to hard (A is easy ... D is hard). In the case of perfect scales, person scores assigned to each response pattern exactly identify the specific items answered correctly or incorrectly. No information is lost by replacing item response patterns with person scores. For example, a person with a score of 3 and a perfect response pattern [1110] is expected to respond correctly to the three easiest items (A, B, and C), and incorrectly to the hardest item (D). A four-item test composed of dichotomous items has 16 possible response patterns ($2^4 = 16$). There are five perfect response patterns, and eleven imperfect patterns. The five perfect patterns are shown in the top panel of Table 2.1 with numbers 1 to 5.

Table 2.1 Guttman Scaling: Response patterns for four dichotomous items (A, B, C and D)

		Perfect Guttman Item Patterns			
Index	Person Scores	A Easy	B	C	D Hard
1	4	1	1	1	1
2	3	1	1	1	0
3	2	1	1	0	0
4	1	1	0	0	0
5	0	0	0	0	0
		Imperfect Guttman Item Patterns			
6	3	1	1	0	1
7	3	1	0	1	1
8	3	0	1	1	1
9	2	1	0	1	0
10	2	0	1	1	0
11	2	1	0	0	1
12	2	0	1	0	1
13	2	0	0	1	1
14	1	0	1	0	0
15	1	0	0	1	0
16	1	0	0	0	1

Note. Four dichotomous items yield 16 possible response patterns (2^4). Items are ordered from easy (Item A) to hard (Item D). There are five perfect Guttman patterns (Index numbers 1 to 5), and 11 imperfect Guttman patterns (Index numbers from 1 to 16).

The 11 imperfect patterns are shown in the bottom panel of Table 2.1 with index numbers 6 to 16. In the case of imperfect Guttman patterns, person scores do not map invariantly to a particular item pattern and vice versa. For example, a person score of one on an imperfect scale can be obtained by three possible response patterns: [0100], [0010], and [0001].

Another way to illustrate a Guttman scale is to use operating characteristic functions that are defined as showing the probabilistic relationship between a latent variable and responses (Samejima, 1983). Two subtypes of operating characteristic functions can be defined that focus either on item response functions or person response functions. This revisits the idea of duality in measurement (Mosier, 1940, 1941). Scales and variable maps can be represented in graphical form as a line with items ordered from easy to hard, and persons ordered from low to high. As pointed out earlier, this line reflects the latent variable that defines the construct being measured. Item characteristic functions can be used to show the expected or ideal relationship between the

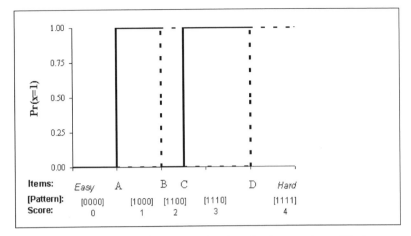

Figure 2.1   Illustrative item characteristic functions for Guttman Items (Ideal, deterministic model).

latent variable being measured and the probability of correctly answering an item. Guttman scales are considered deterministic models (Torgerson, 1958). Deterministic models specify the exact responses that are expected in each cell, while probabilistic models allow the responses to vary between 0 and 1 for dichotomous scores (x = 0, 1). Guttman items yield the distinctive triangular pattern of responses shown in Table 2.1, and also the distinctive stair-step pattern in Figure 2.1.

The x-axis in Figure 2.1 represents the latent variable with items A to D ordered from easy to hard. The items are rank ordered, and there is no requirement that the x-axis have equal intervals. The y-axis represents the probability of responding with a correct answer to each item. For example, a person located on the x-axis between items B and C is expected to answer Items A and B correctly (probability is 1.00) and items C and D incorrectly (probability is .00); this yields a score of 2 and a perfect response pattern [1100]. These distinctive step functions also serve to define a Guttman scale.

In addition to item response functions, there are also operating characteristics functions for person responses within the context of ideal Guttman scales. These scales yield "perfect conjoint transitivity" (Wright, 1997, p. 37).

> If a person endorses a more extreme statement, he should endorse all less extreme statements if the statements are to be considered a scale ... We shall call a set of items of common content a scale if a person with a higher rank than another person is just as high or higher on every item than the other person. (Guttman, 1950, p. 62)

Person response functions can also be shown graphically as step functions that would be mirror images of the step functions of item response functions.

In a perfect Guttman scale, the property of transitivity is invariant over persons. Guttman recognized that the scalability of a set of items may not be invariant over different groups of persons. This becomes a very important issue because if the items are not invariant over groups, then it is not possible to compare them.

> If a universe is scalable for one population but not for another population or forms a scale in a different manner, we cannot compare the two populations in degree and say that one is higher or lower on the average than another with respect to the universe. (Guttman, 1944, p. 150)

This concern with item invariance across groups appears within modern measurement in the form of differential item functioning and measurement invariance. It also highlights the idea of falsifiability, and the importance of goodness-of-fit as evidence regarding whether or not invariant measurement has been achieved with a particular set of items and group of persons.

What Are Rasch Models?

Rasch proposed a set of measurement models that provide an opportunity to meet the five requirements of invariant measurement (Rasch, 1960/1980). There are a variety of specific Rasch models that are described in later chapters. The family of Rasch models includes ideal-type models for dichotomous, polytomous, partial credit, rating scale, and many-facet data. Rasch models have also been developed for Poisson counts, Binomial trials, multidimensional assessments, and multilevel data forms. In this section, the focus is on the dichotomous Rasch model.

Andrich (1985) has made a strong and persuasive case for viewing the Rasch model as a probabilistic realization of a Guttman scale. The Rasch model for dichotomous data can be used to model the probability of dichotomous responses as a logistic function of item difficulty and person location on the latent variable. The probability of a correct response ($x_{ni} = 1$) under the Rasch model can be written as follows:

$$P_{ni1} = \Pr(x_{ni}=1|\theta_n,\delta_i) = \exp(\theta_n - \delta_i)/ [1 + \exp(\theta_n - \delta_i)] \qquad [1]$$

and the probability of an incorrect response ($x_{ni} = 0$)

$$P_{ni0} = \Pr(x_{ni}=0|\theta_n,\delta_i) = 1 / [1 + \exp(\theta_n - \delta_i)] \qquad [2]$$

where x_{ni} is the observed response from person n on item i (0 = incorrect, 1 = correct), θ_n is the location of person n on the latent variable, and δ_i is the difficulty of item i on the same scale. Once estimates of θ_n and δ_i are available, then the probability of each item response and item response pattern can be calculated based on the Rasch model.

If Guttman's model is written within this framework, then Guttman items can be represented as follows for a correct response:

$$P_{ni1} = \Pr(x_{ni} = 1|\theta_n, \delta_i) = 1, \text{ if } \theta_n \geq \delta_i \qquad [3]$$

The form for an incorrect response with Guttman items is:

$$P_{ni0} = \Pr(x_{ni} = 0|\theta_n, \delta_i) = 0, \text{ if } \theta_n < \delta_i. \qquad [4]$$

This reflects the deterministic nature of Guttman items that was illustrated in Figure 2.1. Guttman's requirement of perfect ordering and transitivity appears within the Rasch measurement model as perfect transitivity in the probabilities of ordered item responses.

Table 2.2 displays the relationship between the response patterns of four items based on data from Stouffer and Toby (1951). This is a classic data set that has been re-analyzed with different measurement models by a variety of authors including Andersen (1980), Lazarsfeld and Henry (1968), and Goodman (1975). Table 2.2 uses the Rasch estimates of item difficulties and person locations based on analyses in Engelhard (2008).

The first column in Table 2.2 is an index column. The second column indicates the possible scores on a four-item test ranging from 0 to 4 with Rasch person locations indicated in parentheses. Rasch person locations are not estimated for perfect scores (0 or 4). Procedures are available for imputing values for these scores that will be discussed later. Column 3 lists the 16 (24) possible response patterns for four dichotomous items. The response patterns are organized by person score, and the first response pattern within each person score set represents the ideal Guttman pattern for the score. For example, the ideal Guttman response pattern is [1110] for a score of 3. The next column gives the observed frequencies of these response patterns from Stouffer and Toby (1951).

The expected response patterns for the four items from Stouffer and Toby (1951) are based on the estimated item difficulties and person locations obtained in Engelhard (2008a). Columns 5 to 8 list the four items from easy to hard with cell entries obtained based on the Rasch model in Equation 1. For example, the expected responses in terms of item probabilities are [.86 .54 .51 .09] for a raw score of 2. This expected pattern is the same for all of the observed response patterns that sum to a raw score of 2. In order to illustrate how the probabilities are obtained, we can substitute the person location of −.06 for the raw score of 2 with the difficulty for Item A (−1.89) in Equation 1. The steps in the calculations are illustrated below:

1. $\Pr(x = 1|-.06, -1.89) = \exp(-.06 - (-1.89))/[1 + \exp(-.06 - (-1.89))]$
2. $\Pr(x = 1|-.06, -1.89) = \exp(1.83)/[1 + \exp(1.83)]$
3. $\Pr(x = 1|-.06, -1.89) = 6.23/[7.23]$
4. $\Pr(x = 1|-.06, -1.89) = .86$
   Reminders: $e = 2.718$ and $\exp(n) = e^n \approx 2.718^n$

Table 2.2 Rasch Model: Probabilities of Item Responses for Four Dichotomous Items (A, B, C and D)

Index	*Person Scores* (θ)	*Item Patterns* ABCD	*Observed Frequency*	*Expected Response Pattern for Items (δ)*			
		Four Items	N = 216	A (–1.89) Easy	B (–.20)	C (–.10)	D (2.20) Hard
1	(High) 4	1111	20	–	–	–	–
2	3 (1.52)	1110	38	.97	.85	.84	.34
		1101	9	.97	.85	.84	.34
		1011	6	.97	.85	.84	.34
		0111	2	.97	.85	.84	.34
3	2 (–.06)	1100	24	.86	.54	.51	.09
		1010	25	.86	.54	.51	.09
		0110	7	.86	.54	.51	.09
		1001	4	.86	.54	.51	.09
		0101	2	.86	.54	.51	.09
		0011	1	.86	.54	.51	.09
4	1 (–1.54)	1000	23	.59	.21	.19	.02
		0100	6	.59	.21	.19	.02
		0010	6	.59	.21	.19	.02
		0001	1	.59	.21	.19	.02
5	0 (Low)	0000	42	–	–	–	–

Note. Rasch analysis of Stouffer and Toby Data (1951) with estimated Rasch item difficulties of –1.89, –.20, –.10, and 2.20 logits for items A to D respectively, and estimated Rasch person locations of –1.54, –.06, and 1.52.

Similar calculations can be used to obtain the other probabilities in Table 2.2. It should be noted that the closest match between response patterns and the Rasch probabilities is found with the perfect Guttman patterns in each score group. The details regarding how to obtain estimates of item difficulties and person locations are described in a later chapter.

The item response functions for these four items based on the dichotomous Rasch model are shown in Figure 2.2. The logistic curves with their distinctive s-shape represent the stochastic relationship between the probability of a correct response (x = 1) for each item as a function of theta. Theta is the Greek letter used to represent the location of persons on the latent variable. These

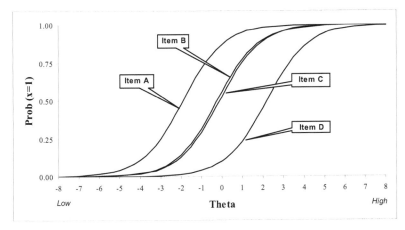

Figure 2.2   Item characteristic functions for Rasch model (ideal, probabilistic model).

can be contrasted with the deterministic structure of the item response functions for Guttman items shown in Figure 2.1.

Item-Invariant Person Measurement

In order to illustrate the duality of invariant measurement, this section provides a detailed example of item-invariant person measurement, while the following section does the same for person-invariant item calibration. The goal of item-invariant person measurement is to develop instruments composed of items that can be used to measure an individual's location on a latent variable that are not dependent on the particular items included in the item sets. In order to illustrate this idea, a variable map is presented in Figure 2.3. This is a variable map for Person A with a location on the latent variable at zero ($\theta_A = 0.00$). There are three sets of items (Sets 1, 2, and 3) with each set composed of four items that vary in difficulty or location on the latent variable. For example, Item Set 1 is composed of four items with the following difficulties: $\delta_{12} = -2.00$, $\delta_{14} = -.50$, $\delta_{15} = .50$ and $\delta_{17} = 1.50$. Based on the Rasch model, persons with locations above the item difficulties are expected to succeed on the items, while persons with locations below the items are expected to fail these items. In Figure 2.3, Column 1 represents the underlying latent variable on the logit scale, Columns 2 to 4 represent the item locations within item sets 1, 2 and 3. Column 5 shows the location of the person on the scale, while the last three columns indicate the responses that Person A made on each of the three item sets. It should be clear in this figure that if the person responds as expected, then Person A's raw score on Item Set 1 is 2 (50% correct), it is 3 on Item Set 2 (75% correct), and it is 1 on Item Set 3 (25% correct). This example demonstrates how total scores defined as number correct or percentage correct score are not invariant over different subsets of items that vary in difficulty.

Logit Scale	Item Difficulties			Person A	Responses		
	Set 1	Set 2	Set 3		Set 1	Set 2	Set 3
5.00							
4.00							
3.00				δ_{38}			0
2.00							
	δ_{17}			δ_{37}	0		0
1.00				δ_{36}			0
	δ_{15}	δ_{25}			0	0	
.00				$\theta_A = 0.00$			
	δ_{14}				1		
-1.00		δ_{23}	δ_{33}		1		1
-2.00	δ_{12}	δ_{22}			1	1	
-3.00		δ_{21}				1	
-4.00							
-5.00							
Raw score					2	3	1
Percent-correct score					50%	75%	25%

Note. Person location on latent variable is fixed ($\theta_A = .00$). Responses and raw scores are dependent on the particular item difficulties on item set s (Sets 1, 2 and 3). Raw scores and percent-correct scores are not invariant over subsets of items.

Figure 2.3　Variable Map for Person A: Item-invariant person measurement ($\theta_A = .00$).

Person-Invariant Item Calibration

Turning now to the other aspect of invariant measurement, the goal of person-invariant item calibration is to develop a set of calibrated items that can be used for measurement that are not dependent on the particular persons or subsets of examinees used to calibrate the item sets. The variable map can also be used to illustrate person-invariant item calibration. In Figure 2.4, a variable map for Item One with a location on the latent variable at $-.50$ logits ($\delta_1 = -.50$) is shown. There are three groups of persons (Groups A, B, and C) with each group having five persons that vary in their location on the latent variable. For example, Group A is composed on five persons with the following locations: $\theta_{A1} = -3.00$, $\theta_{A2} = -1.50$, $\theta_{A3} = -.50$, $\theta_{A4} = .50$ and $\theta_{A5} = 2.50$. Based on the Rasch model, persons with locations above the item difficulties are expected to succeed on the items, while persons with locations below the

Logit Scale	Person Locations			Item One	Responses		
	Group A	Group B	Group C		Group A	Group B	Group C
5.00							
4.00			θ_{C5}				1
3.00							
	θ_{A5}				1		
2.00			θ_{C4}				1
1.00							
	θ_{A4}		θ_{C3}		1		1
.00			θ_{C2}				1
	θ_{A3}	θ_{B5}		$\delta_1 = -.50$	1	1	
-1.00							
	θ_{A2}				0		
-2.00		θ_{B4}	θ_{C1}			0	0
-3.00	θ_{A1}	θ_{B3}			0	0	
-4.00		θ_{B2}				0	
-5.00		θ_{B1}				0	
Item Score					3	1	4
P-value (percent correct)					60%	20%	80%

Note. Item location on latent variable is fixed ($\delta_1 = -.50$). Responses and item scores are dependent on the particular person groups (Groups A, B, and C). Item scores and p-values are not invariant over subgroups of persons.

Figure 2.4   Variable Map for Item One: Person-invariant item calibration ($\delta_1 = -.50$).

items are expected to fail these items. In Figure 2.4, Column 1 represents the underlying latent variable on the logit scale, Columns 2 to 4 represent the person locations within Groups A, B, and C. Column 5 shows the location of the item on the scale, while the last three columns indicate the responses that persons made on Item One. If a person responds as expected, then each person is expected to succeed on Item One if their location is below the item, and to fail if their location is below Item One. The difficulty of Item One for Groups A, B, and C yield p-values respectively of 60%, 20%, and 80%. It is clear that percentage correct or p-values are not sample-independent estimates of item difficulty. Item scores and p-values are not invariant over person groups. As was the case for item-invariant measurement, Rasch models can provide a theoretical framework that adjusts for differences in person groups using item response functions. It should be stressed that both item-invariant person measurement and person-invariant item calibration are based on an ideal-type perspective on measurement. The results presented in these two sections hold exactly based on the parameterization of the dichotomous Rasch model. The purpose has been to illustrate how invariant measurement appears for both persons and items within the theoretical framework of the Rasch model under ideal circumstances.

Discussion and Summary

This chapter focused on introducing invariant measurement based on the ideal-type views of measurement embodied in Guttman scaling and Rasch measurement models. As suggested in the opening quotes regarding Einstein's research work, the quest for invariance has been a cornerstone of science. Invariant measurement can be viewed as stressing similar requirements for measurement within the social, behavioral, and health sciences.

Both Guttman scaling and Rasch models provide measurement frameworks that are intuitively appealing using ideal-type models for conceptualizing aspects of invariant measurement. As pointed out by Cliff (1983) the

> Guttman scale is one of the very clearest examples of a good idea in all of psychological measurement. Even with an unsophisticated—but intelligent—consumer of psychometrics, one has only to show him a perfect scale and the recognition is almost instantaneous, "Yes, that's what I want." (p. 284)

Guttman scaling is important because it lays out in a very obvious way many of the issues and requirements that are necessary for the development of a scale that meets the requirements of invariant measurement. Even though his requirements for a perfect scale are embedded within a deterministic framework, Andrich (1985) has shown how a probabilistic model based on Rasch measurement theory (Rasch, 1960/80) can achieve these theory-based requirements. Andrich (1985) has also pointed out the close connections between Guttman's deterministic model and Rasch's probabilistic model.

> technical parallels between the SLM [simple logistic model, dichotomous Rasch model] and the Guttman scale are not a coincidence. The connections arise from the same essential conditions required in both, including the requirement of invariance of scale and location values with respect to each other. (Andrich, 1988, p. 40)

In Guttman's ideal-type model for measurement, responses are simply a function of person and item locations on the construct. In the real world, responses are not deterministic, and there is a stochastic element as well as other sources of construct-irrelevant variation that may affect responses in addition to person and item locations on the latent variable. The value of Rasch models as probabilistic versions of Guttman scales have led to comments, such as this one by Loevinger (1965): "Rasch (1960) has devised a truly new approach to psychometric problems ... [that yields] non-arbitrary measures" (p. 151).

This chapter began with a brief description of measurement as a process for locating both persons and items on a latent variable. Variable maps were introduced as visual displays for conveying in a concrete fashion the latent variable. Next, the philosophical issues underlying invariant measurement were presented. In particular, the importance of stressing the requirements of measurement based on ideal-types leads to a focus on creating data structures that meet these requirements in order to gain the benefits of invariant measurement. This view is contrasted with a statistical perspective that stresses fitting models to extant data. The duality of measurement as combining aspects of both item calibration and the measurement of persons on a latent variable was also introduced. The structure of measurement data was presented with a simple deterministic model based the ideal measurement scales conceptualized by Louis Guttman. After the introduction of Guttman scaling and the Rasch model for dichotomous data, the point was stressed that the Rasch model can be viewed as a stochastic or probabilistic version of Guttman's deterministic scaling model. Person and item response functions were introduced next with two simple examples of invariant measurement provided to illustrate item-invariant person measurement and person-invariant item calibration.

Chapter 3

Rasch Models

This chapter describes four versions of the Rasch model that can meet the five requirements of invariant measurement. The specific models are the Dichotomous model, two polytomous models for rating-scale data (Partial Credit and Rating Scale models), and the Many Facet model. Wright and Masters (1982) describe a family of Rasch models that includes two other Rasch models (the binomial trials model and the Poisson counts model) that are not included here. There are several other Rasch models available including a linear logistic test model (Fischer, 1997), a random coefficients multinomial logit model (Adams & Wilson, 1996), as well as a multidimensional version of the Rasch model (Adams, Wilson, & Wang, 1997). These three models are not included in this chapter.

Table 3.1 provides an overview of the models examined in this chapter. It should be stressed that the Rasch measurement models described in this chapter are ideal-type representations of the relationships among responses (dichotomous, polytomous), person locations and item locations on a latent variable. This chapter shows how the generalized item parameter (δ_{ij}) can be defined in different ways to reflect different members of the family of Rasch models.

This family of Rasch models can be viewed as ideal types related to the methodological approach proposed for social science research by the German sociologist Max Weber (Coser, 1977). In essence, these ideal types represent Rasch models that meet the requirements of invariant measurement completely because of the way they are defined. This is similar to the underlying principles of Guttman scaling with an a priori statement of the requirements of sound measurement, and then the development of a scaling model to meet these requirements. Rasch models can be viewed as probabilistic versions of Guttman scales (Andrich, 1985). Although Guttman scaling models are deterministic and Rasch measurement models are probabilistic, they both exemplify the notion of an ideal measurement situation that researchers seek to attain in practical assessment situations. Judgments regarding how well actual data meet the requirements of these ideal models revolve around issues of model-data fit that are addressed in a later chapter. Again, the equations

Table 3.1   General Form of the Operating Characteristic Function for Defining a Family of Rasch Measurement Models

Operating characteristic function:

Probability of moving from category k-1 to k	$\phi_{nmik} = \dfrac{P_{nmik}}{P_{nmik-1} + P_{nmik}} = \dfrac{\exp(\theta_n - \delta_{mik})}{1 + \exp(\theta_n - \delta_{mik})}$

Rasch Models:

δ_{mik} defined as	δ_i	Dichotomous Model
	δ_{ik}	Partial Credit Model
	$\delta_i + \tau_k$	Rating Scale Model
	δ_{mik}	Many Facet Model

Note. These are the specific Rasch models discussed in this book.

and figures in this chapter are ideal representations of Rasch models that are perfect in the sense of meeting all the requirements of invariant measurement. These measurement models form the basis for constructing variable maps that provide clear and simple visual representations of the latent variable of interest in terms of the locations of persons and items.

In the next section, the concept of operating characteristic functions is introduced. Next, the Dichotomous Rasch model (Rasch, 1960/1980) is presented. Following this section, the Partial Credit model (Masters, 1982) and Rating Scale model (Andrich, 1978a, b) are introduced for use with polytomous data collected in the form of rating scales with ordered categories. The next section provides a description of the Many Facet model (Linacre, 1994, 2007) that can be used for extending the Rasch model to include an additional facet, such as raters. Finally, key points and themes are highlighted in the discussion and summary section.

Operating Characteristic Functions

The ideas presented in this chapter are organized around the concept of an operating characteristic function. Operating characteristic (OC) functions provide a useful way to conceptualize the relationship of responses with person and item locations on the latent variable. The concept of OC functions has been described by Samejima (1983). Samejima (1983) offered the following definition: "The operating characteristic of the item response on the discrete response level is the conditional probability function of the item response, give the latent [variable]" (p. 160). Rasch (1960/1980) proposed using the cumulative distribution function of the logistic distribution as the OC functions for modeling dichotomous data. This can be written as

$$\Psi\left(x\right) = \frac{\exp(x)}{1+\exp(x)} \qquad [1]$$

with x defined as a variable that can take on values between $-\infty$ to $+\infty$, exp represents exponents to base 2.718, and the symbol (Ψ) represents the logistic distribution function. The obtained values from this function vary between 0 and 1. For example, if x = 0, then the exp(0) = 1, 1+ exp(0) = 2, and therefore Ψ(0) = .50. Within the context of Rasch measurement, x is defined as the difference or distance between person and item locations on a latent variable and the values of the function are defined as the probability of a correct or positive responses (x =1). This can be written as

$$\phi_{ni} = P_{ni} = \Psi\left(\theta_n - \delta_i\right) \qquad [2]$$

where P_{ni} is the conditional probability of a correct response given the differences between the location of persons (θ_n) and items (δ_i). This logistic function can also be used to define a person response function. If a particular person is selected, such as Person A, then the OC function defines a person response function that represents the probability of Person A succeeding on a set of L ordered items. This can be written as

$$\phi_{Ai} = P_{Ai} = \Psi\left(\theta_A - \delta_i\right) \qquad [3]$$

Figure 3.1 presents several illustrative operating characteristic functions. Panel A shows graphically Equation 3 for Person A. The probability of a correct response (x = 1) decreases as the difficulty of the items (δ_i) increases. Panel C presents the person response function for an incorrect response (x = 0) with the probability of an incorrect response increasing as the difficulty of the items increase. Figure 3.2 presents five person response functions that vary in location on the latent variable from a low for Person A ($\theta_A = -2.00$ logits) to a high for Person E ($\theta_E = 2.50$ logits).

Conversely, if a particular item is selected, such as Item 1, then the OC function defines an item response function. Item response functions as shown in Equation 4 have also been called item characteristic functions,

$$\phi_{n1} = P_{n1} = \Psi\left(\theta_n - \delta_1\right) \qquad [4]$$

item characteristic curves, and trace lines. Item response functions for Item 1 are shown in Figure 3.1. Panel B illustrates how the probability of a correct response on Item 1 increases as the location of persons on the latent variable increases. Panel D shows the mirror image of Panel B, and represents the probability of an incorrect response. Figure 3.3 presents four item response functions that vary in location on the latent variable from an easy item (Item 1 with $\delta_1 = -2.50$ logits) to a difficult item (Item 4 with $\delta_4 = 2.00$ logits).

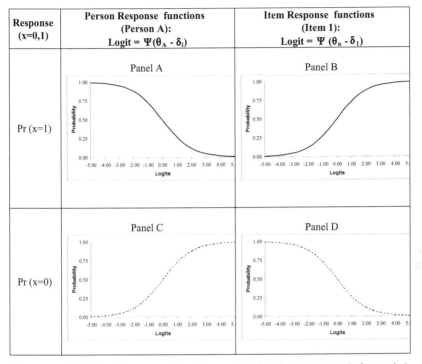

Response (x=0,1)	Person Response functions (Person A): Logit = $\Psi(\theta_A - \delta_i)$	Item Response functions (Item 1): Logit = $\Psi(\theta_n - \delta_1)$
Pr (x=1)	Panel A	Panel B
Pr (x=0)	Panel C	Panel D

Note. x represents the observed response or rating with x equal to 0 for an incorrect response (or lower rating) and 1 for a correct response (or higher rating). θ is the location of the person on the latent variable, and δ is the location of the item on the latent variable.

Figure 3.1   Illustrative operating characteristics functions for the Dichotomous Rasch Model (Person A and Item 1).

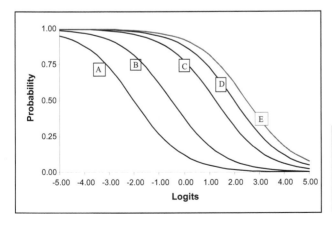

Persons	θ
Person A =	-2.00
Person B =	-0.50
Person C =	1.25
Person D +	2.00
Person E =	2.50

Figure 3.2   Five Rasch Person Response Functions (Ordered from Persons A to Person E).

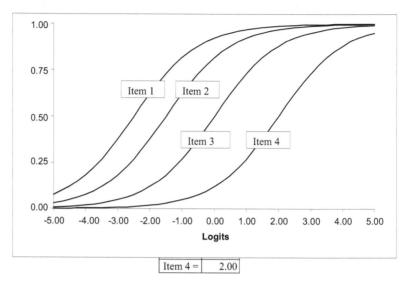

It should be pointed out that for the dichotomous case (x = 0, 1), the operating characteristic function and item response function have the same form. This distinction becomes important when modeling responses to polytomous data with ordered categories (x = 0, 1, ..., m). In the polytomous case with more than two categories, the dichotomous Rasch model can be used to model the probability of moving across adjacent ordered categories: 0 to 1 (no, yes), 1 to 2 (no, yes), 2 to 3 (no, yes) etc. As pointed out by Samejima (1983), "when an item is scored into more than two graded response categories, the operating characteristic must be specified for each item score category" (p. 160). OC functions also play a role in distinguishing between parametric and nonparametric item response theory (IRT) models. Parametric IRT models specify the form of the OC functions, and the task of the researcher is to estimate the item and person parameters for this particular form of the model. In the case of nonparametric IRT models, the researcher is trying to estimate the overall form of the OC functions without any prior theory or model regarding its structure.

Dichotomous Rasch Model

Georg Rasch introduced a Rasch model for dichotomous responses (x = 0,1) during the 1950s. The operating characteristic function for this model is shown in Table 3.2. In the left column, the general form of the OC functions for the Rasch models is shown. Next, Table 3.2 shows the specialization of the general OC functions for the dichotomous Rasch model:

Table 3.2   Dichotomous Rasch Model (Responses in two ordered categories (x = 0, 1)

Operating Characteristic Function	Category Response Function

General Form

$$\phi_{nmik} = \frac{P_{nmik}}{P_{nmik-1} + P_{nmik}} = \frac{\exp(\theta_n - \delta_{mik})}{1 + \exp(\theta_n - \delta_{mik})} \qquad \pi_{nmik} = \frac{\exp\left[\displaystyle\sum_{j=0}^{k}(\theta_n - \delta_{mik})\right]}{\displaystyle\sum_{r=0}^{m_i}\exp\left[\displaystyle\sum_{j=0}^{r}(\theta_n - \delta_{mik})\right]}$$

Dichotomous Rasch Model (Item Response Functions: x=1 for correct response or higher rating)

$$\phi_{ni1} = \frac{P_{ni1}}{P_{ni0} + P_{ni1}} = \frac{\exp(\theta_n - \delta_{i1})}{1 + \exp(\theta_n - \delta_{i1})} \qquad \pi_{ni1} = \frac{\exp\left[\displaystyle\sum_{j=0}^{1}(\theta_n - \delta_{ij})\right]}{\displaystyle\sum_{r=0}^{1}\exp\left[\displaystyle\sum_{j=0}^{r}(\theta_n - \delta_{ij})\right]}$$

$$\phi_{ni1} = \frac{P_{ni1}}{1} = \frac{\exp(\theta_n - \delta_{i1})}{1 + \exp(\theta_n - \delta_{i1})} \qquad \pi_{ni1} = \frac{\exp(\theta_n - \delta_{i1})}{1 + \exp(\theta_n - \delta_{i1})}$$

$$\phi_{ni1} = \frac{\exp(\theta_n - \delta_{i1})}{1 + \exp(\theta_n - \delta_{i1})} \qquad \pi_{ni1} = \frac{\exp(\theta_n - \delta_{i1})}{1 + \exp(\theta_n - \delta_{i1})}$$

Note. P_{ni1} is the conditional probability of scoring 1 on item i, P_{ni0} is the conditional probability of scoring 0 on item i, θ_n is the location of person n on the latent variable, and δ_{i1} is the location on the latent variable where the probability of responding in adjacent categories, 0 and 1, is equal. For the dichotomous case δ_{i1} is defined as the difficulty of item i. The operating characteristic function and the category response function are the same for dichotomous items as shown in the last row of the table.

$$\phi_{ni1} = \frac{\exp(\theta_n - \delta_{i1})}{1 + \exp(\theta_n - \delta_{i1})} \qquad [5]$$

Equation 5 represents the conditional probability of person n on item i responding with a correct response (x = 1) or receiving a rating of 1. As pointed out earlier, the dichotomous OC functions can be used to represent both person and item response functions. The person location (θ) is fixed for the person response function, while the item difficulty or item location (δ) is fixed for the item response function.

In addition to considering the operating characteristic function, it is important to introduce the concept of a category response function. Category response functions (CRFs) directly represent the conditional probability of responding in each ordered category. The general form of the CRF for the dichotomous Rasch model is shown in column 2 of Table 3.2. The specialization of the CRF to the case of the dichotomous Rasch model is also shown in Table 3.2. The CRF for the dichotomous Rasch model is:

$$\pi_{ni1} = \frac{\exp(\theta_n - \delta_{i1})}{1 + \exp(\theta_n - \delta_{i1})} \qquad [6]$$

Table 3.2 shows that the operating characteristic and category response functions are the same for the dichotomous Rasch model. The distinction between these two functions becomes important in generalizing the dichotomous Rasch model for rating scales and other ordered response data that is collected in two or more categories.

Table 3.3 presents the dichotomous Rasch model in log-odds form. This form highlights the roles of the person (q) and item locations (d) in the model. It illustrates how the Rasch model can be viewed as a type of logistic regression with the log odds as the dependent variable and the two facets in the model (person and item location on the latent variable) viewed as independent variables that predict the probability of moving from one category to the next category. The dichotomous Rasch model is appropriate for modeling a variety of scores and ratings that can be scored as 0 or 1, such as the responses to multiple-choice items (0 = incorrect, 1 = correct) or ratings (0 = not present, 1 = present).

Table 3.3   Dichotomous Rasch Models in Log-odd Form

Conditional probability: Pr (x=1)	$\phi_{ni1} = \dfrac{\exp(\theta_n - \delta_{i1})}{1 + \exp(\theta_n - \delta_{i1})}$
Conditional probability: Pr (x=0)	$\phi_{ni0} = \dfrac{1}{1 + \exp(\theta_n - \delta_{i1})}$
Odds: Pr (x=1)/ Pr (x=0)	$\dfrac{\phi_{ni1}}{\phi_{ni0}} = \exp(\theta_n - \delta_i)$
Log-odds of operating characteristic function[1]	$Ln\dfrac{\phi_{ni1}}{\phi_{ni0}} = \theta_n - \delta_i$

1. Operating characteristic and category response functions are the same for the dichotomous Rasch model

Polytomous Rasch Models

There are a variety of Rasch models that can be used to analyze ordered rating scale data. Rating scale data are defined as person responses that are scored in two or more ordered categories. Rating scale data represent the most common formats for collecting information from persons or raters. The basic idea that motivates the use of Rasch models for rating scale data is that the scoring of categories with ordered integers (0,1, ..., m) may be based on the unexamined assumption that the categories define equal intervals on the latent variable. This assumption may not be justified when empirical information is examined. Rasch models provide a framework to explicitly examine this assumption, and to parameterize the intervals that define the categories without the assumption that the categories are of equal size. The specific Rasch models described in this section on polytomous Rasch models are the Partial Credit model (Masters, 1982) and Rating Scale model (Andrich, 1978b).

Rating scales are among the most common formats for collecting observations in the behavioral, social and health sciences. A rating scale for item i provides the opportunity for a person to select a score X in m_i +1 ordered categories (x = 0, 1, ... , m_i). For example, the person might be indicating his or her attitude using a Likert Scale (0 = Strongly Disagree, 1 = Disagree, 2 = Uncertain, 3 = Strongly Agree, 4 = Agree) or a rater might be judging the quality of student writing (0 = novice, 1 = proficient, 2 = accomplished). If there are two response categories (0 = incorrect, 1 = correct), then the ratings yield dichotomous data. If there are three or more categories, then the ratings yield polytomous data. Higher ratings are intended to indicate a higher location on the latent variable with the latent variable representing an unobservable construct or trait. The goal of measurement is to locate both persons and items on this underlying latent variable in order to define a measuring instrument.

One of the central problems in measurement is the development of models that can connect person measures and item calibrations in a meaningful way to represent a latent variable. In this book, the variable map is an operational definition of the latent variable. The basic idea that motivates the use of Rasch models for rating scale data is that the scoring of ordered categories with ordered integers (0,1, ..., m) implies that there are equal intervals between the thresholds that define the categories. In other words, the distances between 0 to 1, 1 to 2, 2 to 3, and so on, are assumed be equal with units of 1.0. This assumption may or may not be justified for a particular data set. Rasch models provide a framework to explicitly examine this assumption, and to parameterize the category coefficients without this assumption. Specifically, Rasch models for rating scale data are used to model category response functions that link the probability of a specific rating or score with person measures and a set of characteristics reflecting item and category calibrations. The category response functions represent the conditional probability of obtaining a score of x on item i as a function of a person's location on the latent variable (q). The general form of the OC functions can be written as follows:

$$\phi_{ni1} = \frac{P_{ni1}}{P_{ni0} + P_{ni1}} = \frac{\exp(\theta_n - \delta_{i1})}{1 + \exp(\theta_n - \delta_{i1})} \qquad [7]$$

for x = 0, 1, ..., m. The Rasch models for rating scale data vary in terms of how they define the operating characteristic functions for the difficulty of moving across adjacent ordered categories. As pointed out earlier for the dichotomous case, the operating characteristic functions are defined as a set of dichotomous models that determine the probability of moving from category k–1 to k.

It should be noted that there are several different ways to categorize models for analyzing rating scale data. In this book, the Rasch models described are unidimensional models for ordered categories. Following Embretson and Reise (2000), these models can be viewed as direct models for ordered polytomous data. Direct models focus directly on estimating category response functions, while the indirect models require two steps that involve first estimating the operating characteristic functions and then estimating the category response functions as a second step. Several indirect models have been proposed for modeling rating scale data. Some examples of these models are the Generalized Partial Credit model (Muraki, 1992, 1997), the Graded Response model (Samejima, 1969, 1997), and the Generalized Graded Response model (Muraki, 1990). See Engelhard (2005a) for a detailed description of these non-Rasch models for rating scale data. The parameterizations of the indirect models do not meet the requirements of invariant measurement as defined in this book. This distinction between direct and indirect models has been labeled divide-by-total and difference models by Thissen and Steinberg (1986).

The equations used to define the dichotomous Rasch model can be presented graphically. In each figure, the x-axis is a logit scale representing the difference between theta values (θ) that represent the location of persons and delta values (δ) representing the location of items or generalized items on the latent variable. The y-axis is the conditional probability of responding in a particular category as a function of the item and category parameters and the q location of each person.

Partial Credit Model

The Partial Credit (PC) model is a unidimensional model for ratings in two or more ordered categories. The PC model is a Rasch model, and therefore provides the opportunity to realize a variety of desirable measurement characteristics related to invariant measurement, such as separability of person and item parameters, sufficient statistics for parameters in the model (Rasch, 1977, 1960/1980), item-invariant measurement of persons and person-invariant calibration of items. When good model-data fit is obtained, then the PC model, as well as other Rasch models, yields invariant measurement (Engelhard,

1994b). The PC model is a straightforward generalization of the Rasch model for dichotomous data applied to pairs of increasing adjacent response categories for ordered rating scale data. The reader should recall that the RS model is designed for rating scales that have the same number and structure of categories across items, while the PC models is designed for rating scales that have variation in the number and usage of categories across items.

As was presented earlier, the Rasch model for dichotomous data can be written as:

$$\phi_{ni1} = \frac{P_{ni1}}{P_{ni0} + P_{ni1}} = \frac{\exp(\theta_n - \delta_{i1})}{1 + \exp(\theta_n - \delta_{i1})} \qquad [8]$$

where P_{i1} is the conditional probability of scoring 1 on item i, P_{i0} is the probability of scoring 0 on item i, θ is the location of the person on the latent variable, and δ_{i1} is the location on the latent variable where the probability of responding in adjacent categories, 0 and 1, is equal. For the dichotomous case δ_{i1} is defined as the difficulty of item i. Equation 8 represents the operating characteristics function for the PC model. When the data are collected with more than two response categories, then the operating characteristic function can be generalized as

$$\phi_{nik} = \frac{P_{nik}}{P_{nik-1} + P_{nik}} = \frac{\exp(\theta_n - \delta_{ik})}{1 + \exp(\theta_n - \delta_{ik})} \qquad [9]$$

where P_{ik} is the probability of scoring k on item i, P_{ik-1} is the probability of scoring k–1 on item i, θ_n is the location of the person on the construct, and δ_{ik} is the location on the construct where the probability of responding in adjacent categories, k–1 and k is equal.

The category response function (CRF) for the PC model is:

$$\pi_{nij} = \frac{\exp\left[\sum_{j=0}^{k}(\theta_n - \delta_{ij})\right]}{\sum_{r=0}^{m_i}\exp\left[\sum_{j=0}^{r}(\theta_n - \delta_{ij})\right]}, \qquad x_i = 0, 1, \ldots, m_i \qquad [10]$$

where $\sum_{j=0}^{0}(\theta - \delta_{ij}) = 0$. The δ_{ij} parameter is interpreted as the intersection between the two consecutive categories where the probabilities of responding in the adjacent categories is equal. The δ_{ij} term is described as a step difficulty by Masters and Wright (1977). Embretson and Reise (2000) have suggested calling the δ_{ij} term a category-intersection parameter. It is important to recognize that the item parameter δ_{ij} represents the location on the latent variable where a person has the same probability of responding in categories k and k–1. These conditional probabilities for adjacent categories are expected to increase, but they are not necessarily ordered from low to high on the latent variable (θ). By defining the item parameters locally, it is possible to verify that persons are using the categories as expected. See Andrich (1978b) for a detailed description of the substantive interpretation of disordered item category parameters.

The Partial Credit model is shown in Figure 3.4. The OC function is shown graphically in the first column, while the CRfunction is shown in the second column. As the category parameters δ_{ix} become closer together (comparing Panels A and B versus Panels C and D), then the probability of being in the middle category decreases.

Rating Scale Model

The Rating Scale (RS) model is another unidimensional Rasch model that can be used to analyze ratings in two or more ordered categories. The RS model, as was the case for the PC model, is a member of the Rasch family of models, and therefore shares the desirable measurement characteristics related to invariant measurement. The RS model is similar to the PC model, but the RS model was developed to analyze rating scale data with a common or fixed number of response categories across a set of items designed to measure a unidimensional construct or latent variable. The PC model does not require the same number of categories for each rating scale item. Likert scales are a prime example of this type of format for rating scales with a fixed number of response categories that are common for all the items in the instrument. For items with the same number of response categories, the RS model decomposes the category parameter, δ_{ij} , from the PC model into two parameters: a location parameter δ_i that reflects item difficulty and a category parameter τ_j . In other words, the δ_{ij} parameter in the PC model is consists of two components, $\delta_{ij} = (\delta_i + \tau_j)$ where δ_i are the locations of the items on the latent variable and the τ_j are the category parameters across items. The category-coefficient parameters are considered equivalent across items for the RS model. The OC function for the RS model is

$$\phi_{nik} = \frac{P_{nik}}{P_{nik-1} + P_{nik}} = \frac{\exp(\theta_n - (\delta_i + \tau_k))}{1 + \exp(\theta_n - (\delta_i + \tau_k))} \qquad [11]$$

where P_{ik} is the probability of scoring k on item i, P_{ik-1} is the conditional probability of scoring k–1 on item i, θ_n is the location of the person on the construct, δ_i are the location of the items on the construct, and τ_k is the location on the construct where the probability of responding in adjacent categories, k–1 and 1, is equal across items. The τ_k parameter has also been called the centralized threshold. The CRFs for the RS model is

$$\pi_{nij} = \frac{\exp\left[\sum_{j=0}^{k}(\theta_n - (\delta_i + \tau_k))\right]}{\sum_{r=0}^{mi}\exp\left[\sum_{j=0}^{r}(\theta_n - (\delta_i + \tau_k))\right]}, \qquad x = 0, 1, \ldots, m \qquad [12]$$

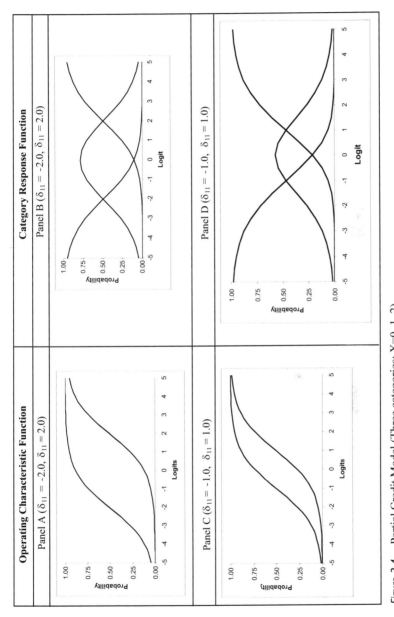

Figure 3.4   Partial Credit Model (Three categories: X=0, 1, 2).

where $\sum_{j=0}^{0} \theta - (\delta_i + \tau_k) \equiv 0$. For the RS model, the shapes of the OC functions and CRFs across items are the same, while the location varies. Both the RS model and PC model are equivalent to the dichotomous Rasch model when the rating scale data are collected in two ordered response categories. The OC and CR functions are summarized in Table 3.4.

The Rating Scale model is shown in Figure 3.5. The OC function is shown graphically in the first column, while the CR function is shown in the second column. The RS model in Figure 3.5 illustrates that even though item locations change ($\delta_1 = 0$, $\delta_2 = 1$), the rating structure is modeled to be constant across items ($\tau_{11} = \tau_{12} = -0.5$, $\tau_{21} = \tau_{22} = 0.5$). This is shown in Panels A and B as compared to Panels C and D where the overall difficulty of the item has increased by one logit ($\delta_1 = 0$ to $\delta_2 = 1$).

Table 3.4   Summary of Rasch Models

Operating Characteristic Function	*Category Response Function*
General Form	
$\phi_{nmik} = \dfrac{P_{nmik}}{P_{nmik-1}+P_{nmik}} = \dfrac{\exp(\theta_n - \delta_{mik})}{1+\exp(\theta_n - \delta_{mik})}$	$\pi_{nmik} = \dfrac{\exp\left[\sum_{j=0}^{k}(\theta_n - \delta_{mik})\right]}{\sum_{r=0}^{m_i}\exp\left[\sum_{j=0}^{r}(\theta_n - \delta_{mik})\right]}$
Dichotomous Model	
$\phi_{ni1} = \dfrac{\exp(\theta_n - \delta_{i1})}{1+\exp(\theta_n - \delta_{i1})}$	$\pi_{ni1} = \dfrac{\exp(\theta_n - \delta_{i1})}{1+\exp(\theta_n - \delta_{i1})}$
Partial Credit Model ($k_i = 0,1,...,K_i$)	
$\phi_{nik} = \dfrac{P_{nik}}{P_{nik-1}+P_{nik}} = \dfrac{\exp(\theta_n - \delta_{ik})}{1+\exp(\theta_n - \delta_{ik})}$	$\pi_{nij} = \dfrac{\exp\left[\sum_{j=0}^{k}(\theta_n - \delta_{ij})\right]}{\sum_{r=0}^{m_i}\exp\left[\sum_{j=0}^{r}(\theta_n - \delta_{ij})\right]}$
Rating Scale Model Responses/ratings ($k = 0,1,...K$)	
$\phi_{nik} = \dfrac{P_{nik}}{P_{nik-1}+P_{nik}} = \dfrac{\exp(\theta_n - (\delta_i + \tau_k))}{1+\exp(\theta_n - (\delta_i + \tau_k))}$	$\pi_{nij} = \dfrac{\exp\left[\sum_{j=0}^{k}(\theta_n - (\delta_i + \tau_k))\right]}{\sum_{r=0}^{m_i}\exp\left[\sum_{j=0}^{r}(\theta_n - (\delta_i + \tau_k))\right]}$
Many Facet Model (Responses/ratings: $k= 0,1,...K$)	
$\phi_{nmik} = \dfrac{P_{nmik}}{P_{nmik-1}+P_{nmik}} = \dfrac{\exp(\theta_n - \lambda_m - \delta_i - \tau_k)}{1+\exp(\theta_n - \lambda_m - \delta_i - \tau_k)}$	$\pi_{nmij} = \dfrac{\exp\left[\sum_{j=0}^{k}(\theta - \lambda_m - \delta_i - \tau_k\right]}{\sum_{r=0}^{m_i}\exp\left[\sum_{j=0}^{r}(\theta_n - \lambda_m - \delta_i - \tau_k)\right]}$

Note. See text for definitions of terms.

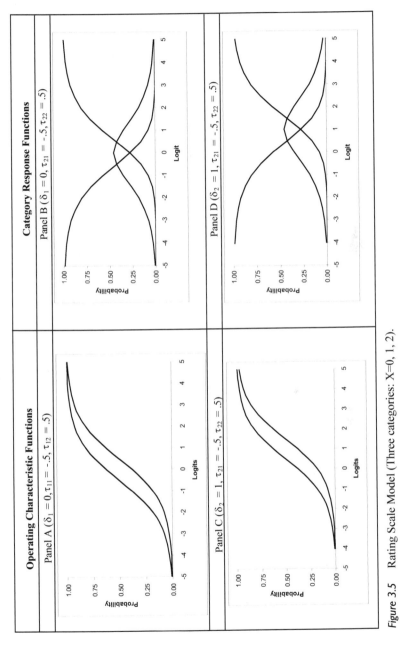

Figure 3.5   Rating Scale Model (Three categories: X=0, 1, 2).

Many Facet Model

The Many Facet (MF) model was originally designed to generalize the Dichotomous, Partial Credit and Rating Scale models for rater-mediated assessments. Rater-mediated (RM) assessments include a variety of performance assessments that require a judge, reader, panelist or assessor to make judgments to assign scores to a person. RM assessments can be contrasted with assessments that score directly the responses of persons to a set of items, such as multiple-choice items. The MF model can also be used to place various designs on items (item subsets) and on persons (person subgroups). The MF model can also be viewed as related to the linear logistic test model (Fischer, 1977). It can be used as an approach to exploratory data analysis similar to fixed effects logistic regression models. MF models have been used to explore grading practices of teachers (Randall & Engelhard, 2009a), writing assessment (Gyagenda & Engelhard, 2009) differential item and person functioning (Engelhard, 2009), and instructional methods (Vogel & Engelhard, 2011).

The OC function for the MF model can be written as:

$$\phi_{nmik} = \frac{P_{nmik}}{P_{nmik-1} + P_{nmik}} = \frac{\exp(\theta_n - \lambda_m - \delta_i - \tau_k)}{1 + \exp(\theta_n - \lambda_m - \delta_i - \tau_k)} \quad [13]$$

and the CR function as follows:

$$\pi_{nmij} = \frac{\exp\left[\sum_{j=0}^{k}(\theta_n - \lambda_m - \delta_i - \tau_k)\right]}{\sum_{r=0}^{mi}\exp\left[\sum_{j=0}^{r}(\theta_n - \lambda_m - \delta_i - \tau_k)\right]} \quad [14]$$

The MF model is essentially an additive linear model that is based on a logistic transformation of observed ratings to a logit or log-odds scale. The logistic transformation of ratios of successive category probabilities (log odds) can be viewed as the dependent variable with various facets, such as writing ability, rater, domain, and task conceptualized as independent variables that influence these log odds. The MF model in log odds format can be written as:

$$Ln\left(\frac{P_{nmik}}{P_{nmik-1}}\right) = \theta_n - \lambda_i - (\delta_i + \tau_k) = \theta_n - \lambda_m - \delta_i - \tau_k \quad [15]$$

where

P_{nmik} = probability of examinee n being rated k on domain i by rater m,
P_{nmik-1} = probability of examinee n being rated k–1 on domain i by rater m,
θ_n = judged location of person n,
λ_m = severity of rater m,
δ_i = judged difficulty of domain i, and
τ_k = judged difficulty of rating category k relative to category k–1.

The rating category coefficient, τ_k, is not considered a facet in the model.

Based on the MF model presented in Equation 15, the probability of examinee n being rated k on domain i for task j by rater m with a rating category coefficient of τ_k is given as

$$\pi_{nmik} = P_{nmik} = exp \; [k \; (\theta_n - \lambda_m - \delta_i - \tau_k) - \delta_i \; \tau_k] \; / \; \gamma \qquad [16]$$

where τ_1 is defined to be zero , and γ is a normalizing factor based on the sum of the numerators. As written in Equation 15, the category coefficients, $\tau_{k,}$ represent a Rating Scale model (Andrich, 1978) with category coefficients fixed across exercises. Analyses using the Partial Credit model (Masters, 1982) with the category coefficients allowed varying across facets can be designated by various subscripts on τ_k. For example, τ_{ik}, would indicate that raters used a different rating scale structure for each domain i, while τ_{mk} would indicate that each rater m used his or her own version of the rating scale.

The MF is a unidimensional model with a single person parameter (location on the latent variable) that represents the object of measurement, and a collection of other facets, such as raters and items. These other facets can be viewed as providing a series of assessment opportunities that yield multiple ratings for each person. For example, if each person is rated by two raters on five items, then there are 10 assessment opportunities that define 10 ratings. As with other Rasch measurement models, the basic requirements of the model are "that the set of people to be measured, and the set of tasks (facets) used to measure them, can each be uniquely ordered in terms respectively of their competence and difficulty" (Choppin, 1987, p. 111). If the data fit the model and this unique ordering related to invariant measurement is realized, then a variety of desirable measurement characteristics can be attained. Some of these measurement characteristics are (a) separability of parameters with sufficient statistics for estimating these parameters, (b) invariant estimates of person, rater and item locations on the latent variable, and (c) equal-interval scales for the measures.

Graphical displays and figures illustrating the MF model in detail are included in later chapters on rater-mediated assessments and other applications of the MF model.

Discussion and Summary

This chapter focused on providing an overview of the Rasch family of models as examples of an ideal-type view of measurement based on a parametric structure that can be viewed as a probabilistic version of Guttman scaling. These models can be used to examine whether or not the five requirements of invariant measurement have met with a particular data set. This family of models is suitable for analyzing ordered response categories that range from dichotomous data (x=0, 1) to polytomous data (x = 0, 1, ..., m) with m categories. All of these models reflect invariant measurement.

Table 3.5 Log-odd Forms of Rasch Models

Dichotomous Model	$Ln \dfrac{P_{ni1}}{P_{ni0}} = \theta_n - \delta_i$
Partial Credit Model	$Ln\left(\dfrac{P_{nik}}{P_{nik-1}}\right) = \theta_n - \delta_{ik}$
Rating Scale Model	$Ln\left(\dfrac{P_{nik}}{P_{nik-1}}\right) = (\theta_n - (\delta_i + \tau_k)) = \theta - \delta_i - \tau_k$

Many Facet Models

Many Facet Partial Credit Model	$Ln\left(\dfrac{P_{nmik}}{P_{nmik-1}}\right) = \theta_n - \lambda_m - \delta_{ik}$
Many Facet Rating Scale Model	$Ln\left(\dfrac{P_{nmik}}{P_{nmik-1}}\right) = \theta_n - \lambda_i - (\delta_i + \tau_k) = \theta_n - \lambda_m - \delta_i - \tau_k$

This chapter focused on four versions of the Rasch model: the Dichotomous model, two polytomous models for rating-scale data (Partial Credit and Rating Scale models), and the Many Facet model. The log-odds format for all of the Rasch models discussed in this chapter are summarized in Table 3.5.

Embretson and Reise (2000), Engelhard (2005), and van der Linden and Hambleton (1997) should be consulted for detailed descriptions of other item response models for rating scale data. The development, comparison and refinement of Rasch models for rating scale data is one of the most active areas in psychometrics. The use of these Rasch models for rater-mediated assessments is developed in later chapters, as well as other applications of the MF model.

All of the Rasch models in this chapter are presented in terms of known parameters, and can be viewed as ideal-type measurement models that meet the five requirements of invariant measurement perfectly. Of course, the challenge is to create operational assessments and variable maps that meet these requirements. This challenge involves obtaining estimates of the parameters in these Rasch models, examining how well-observed data meet the requirements of invariant measurement, and drawing inferences about the locations of both persons and items on the latent variable being created.

Chapter 4

Researcher-Constructed Measures

This chapter focuses on a description of a conceptual framework for guiding the development of researcher-constructed measures. This framework is based on the four building blocks proposed by Mark Wilson (2005). These building blocks are organized around the idea that variable maps define a latent variable in conjunction with an observational design, a set of scoring rules, and a particular measurement model.

Wilson (2005) described an item response modeling approach for constructing measures that provides a detailed description regarding how to develop instruments and scales for measurement. The labels used in this chapter differ slightly from those used by Wilson (2005), although the underlying definitions and descriptions of each building block are conceptually comparable. The building blocks for researcher-constructed measures described in this book are the (1) latent variable, (2) observational design (items), (3) scoring rubric (performance levels), and (4) the Rasch measurement model. The labels used by Wilson (2005) are construct map, items design, outcome space, and measurement model, respectively. Duckor, Draney, and Wilson (2009) should be consulted for an elaboration of Wilson (2005) that includes detailed rubrics to assess the level of understanding of key concepts related to the four building blocks.

The first section of this chapter describes each of these building blocks. Next, two illustrative analyses are provided. The first illustration is based on the measurement of the learning stimulation in the home environments of preschool children (Monsaas & Engelhard, 1996). The second illustration is based on the development of an instrument designed to assess nursing practices related to the five rights for safe administration of medications (Ryan, 2007).

Building Blocks for Researcher-Constructed Measures

Wilson's building blocks provide a conceptual framework for representing the steps needed for the construction of a measure, scale or instrument. The overarching goal is the creation of a variable map of a latent variable, construct or attribute. Figure 4.1 provides a visual representation of these building blocks

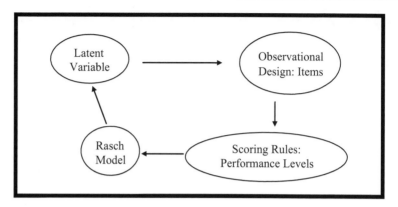

Figure 4.1   Four Building Blocks for Constructing a Variable Map.

with connecting arrows suggesting the interconnections among the various components of the process. It should be stressed that the pathways represented by the arrows are intended to reflect a sequential process, although in some situations the order or steps may be slightly different. It is also typical in the construction of instruments to go through an iterative process that includes information flowing backwards to earlier steps or blocks in a spiral that ultimately leads to improvements in the instrument. The building blocks and the key questions addressed within each block are summarized in Table 4.1.

Each of these building blocks is discussed in the following four sections.

I. Latent Variable: What Is the Latent Variable Being Measured?

The latent variable represents the construct or attribute that is being measured. Variable maps are key visual representations of latent variables. For example, Figure 1.2 in Chapter 1 presented a variable map for measuring the learning stimulation in the home environments of young children. In the development and conceptualization of the latent variable, it is important to consider the underlying continuum in terms of a qualitative order from low to high. Some examples of a qualitative order are fail/pass, less/more, incorrect/correct, no/yes, and disagree/agree. The underlying idea is that if a person responds in a certain way to a stimulus situation (e.g., a multiple-choice item) with ordered responses, then the researcher can draw inferences regarding the person's location on the latent variable based on a combination or summation of these ordered responses. It is hypothesized that the more items that a person responds to in a positive direction (correct answers), then the more likely he or she is to possess more of the latent variable (construct or attribute) being measured by the instrument. This idea of a line with an underlying continuum ordered from low to high reflects the intuitive understanding that most researchers have regarding measurement. It should be noted that variable

Table 4.1   Four Building Blocks and Underlying Questions

Index Building Blocks		*Questions*
1	Latent variable (construct/ attribute)	What is the latent variable being measured?
		1. Is the latent variable unidimensional?
		2. Is there a qualitative order to the latent variable?
		3. Can typical responses that represent locations of less and more be identified on the latent variable?
2	Observational design (items, prompts, or tasks)	What is the plan for collecting structured observations or responses from persons in order to define the latent variable?
		1. What are the construct components (content - knowing) of the latent variable?
		2. What are the distributional components (levels/ categories) ?
		3. What item formats are being used?
3	Scoring rules (answer keys, rubrics, and performance-level descriptors)	How are observations or responses categorized to represent person locations and levels on the latent variable?
		1. What are the definitions for categories or performance levels of persons that are measured?
		2. How are categories scored (scoring scheme)?
4	Rasch model (measurement model)	How are person and item responses or observations mapped onto the latent variable?
		1. Do the locations of persons and items match the order proposed by the researcher in the hypothesized variable map?
		2. How well do the persons and items fit the requirements of the Rasch model?

Goal: Creation of a variable map with locations for both person and items!

maps can be presented in several forms that range from tabular to various graphical displays. The key aspect of the variable map is a visual representation of a line or continuum ranging from low to high with both persons and items mapped onto this continuum.

As shown in Table 4.1, the major underlying question that is addressed with the first building block is: What is the latent variable being measured? Subsidiary questions that should also be addressed are as follows: (a) Is the latent variable unidimensional? (b) Is there a qualitative order to the latent variable? and (c) Can typical responses representing locations of less and more be identified on the latent variable?

2. Observational Design: What Is the Plan for Collecting Structured Observations or Responses from Persons in Order to Define the Latent Variable?

Once the researcher has a general sense of the latent variable, the next step is to design a set of observational or response situations for persons to have the opportunity to exhibit their locations on the construct or attribute. In essence, the researcher creates situations to operationalize and observe person responses in order to locate persons on the latent variable. The observational design lays out the rules for generating item and stimulus situations. It represents a plan for systemically gathering evidence regarding person locations on the latent variable.

Figure 4.2 presents one way to conceptualize observational designs. First of all, the researcher identifies a domain of possible evidence that can be used to define the latent variable.

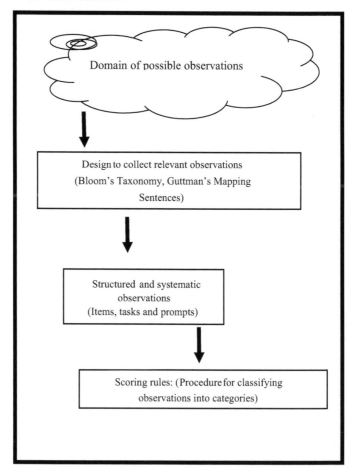

Figure 4.2   Observational design.

This domain has been called a universe of attributes by Guttman (1944, 1950; Engelhard, 2005a). The domain is viewed as a target set of potential items or observations that a scale is designed to represent. This domain has also been called a universe of content. Cronbach, Gleser, Nanda, & Rajaratnam (1972) employ a similar idea when they distinguish between a population of persons and a universe of conditions or observations. Much of the current work on content-related evidence is relevant for validating inferences to a domain based on a sample of person responses or behaviors. Next, a taxonomic or some other theoretical structure is proposed to guide the collection of relevant observations from the domain. The researcher then creates a set of systematic and standardized observational opportunities. These observational opportunities can take the form of test items (multiple-choice, selected-response, or constructed-response), tasks (task shells), and prompts that provide a framework for obtaining responses from persons. Finally, a procedure is developed to classify these observations into categories that represent locations on the latent variable.

In order to illustrate the idea of an observational design, a small example has been constructed. Figure 4.3 presents a set of stars that the researcher wishes to categorize and map onto a scale. Rows one and two present a set of observations that have been collected by the researcher. There are several ways to define a latent variable based on these observations. For example, the

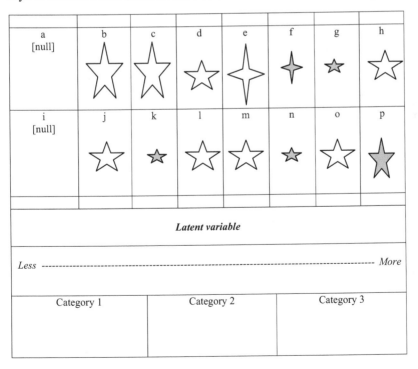

Figure 4.3   Categorize the stars.

researcher might define the latent variable as size with the smallest stars in Category 1 and the largest stars in Category 3:

Category 1(small)	*Category 2(medium)*	*Category 3(large)*
f, g, k, n, p	d, h, j, l, m, o	b, c, e

Or the researcher might decide to map by shading with a null category:

Category 1	*Category 2(no shading)*	*Category 3(shading)*
a, i	b, c, d, e, h, j, l, m, o	f, k, n, p

The category system depends on the latent variable being measured. Other possibilities for classifying the stars might be based on the most valued aesthetic properties or which of the stars was perceived to grant the most wishes. In each case, the categorization system suggests an order of value or worth with Category 1 having the lowest value on the continuum and Category 3 having the highest value. The category order also implies transitivity with Category 3 > Category 2 > Category 1.

Test blueprints and tables of specifications are examples of observational designs that are commonly used to construct educational assessments. Tables of specifications are guided by various taxonomies or classification schemes regarding the content of a specific area of study. One of the first attempts to classify observations is Bloom's taxonomy of educational objectives for the cognitive domain (Bloom, Englehart, Furst, Hill, & Krathwohl, 1956). An example of a table of specifications for a unit on educational measurement is presented in Figure 4.4. The rows represent the content of the measurement unit (What do we want students to know related to the measurement concepts of reliability, validity, and the interpretation of test scores?), while the columns represent the levels of the content unit (What do we want students to be able to do with the content in this measurement unit?).

Other taxonomies have been proposed for the cognitive domain (Biggs & Collis, 1982). Taxonomies have also been proposed for the affective domain (Krathwohl, Bloom, & Masia, 1964). Anderson and Sosniak (1994) provide

	Levels of Bloom's Taxonomy					
Content	Knowledge	Comprehension	Analysis	Application	Synthesis	Evaluation
Reliability	1,2,3		15, 16	18, 19	23	25
Validity	4,5,6,7,8	11,12,13		20, 21		26,27,28
Interpretation of test scores	9,10	14	17	22	24	29, 30

Figure 4.4   Bloom's Taxonomy for an introduction to measurement examination (30 items).

a 40-year retrospective on Bloom's taxonomy, and Guskey (2006) provides a perspective on Bloom's views of the significance of the Taxonomy of Educational Objectives.

Another framework for obtaining structured observations from persons is Guttman's mapping sentences (Borg & Shye, 1995). Guttman's mapping sentences can be used to represent two-facet observational designs, such as Bloom's taxonomy (content x level), but can also be extended to handle observational designs with more facets.

In order to illustrate Guttman mapping sentence, Table 4.2 presents the underlying mapping sentence that guided the research of Jennifer Randall (Randall, 2007; Randall & Engelhard, 2009). This mapping sentence provides the experimental design that guided the generation of items and vignettes, and the collection responses from teachers regarding the grade that they would assign to each student represented by a particular item. Table 4.3 illustrates several sample items describing student descriptions generated from the mapping sentence. The student characteristics are called facets in Guttman's mapping sentences, and the unique combinations of the four student characteristics are called structuples. For example, the first structuple in the table reflects an item designed to represent a student with high ability (3), high achievement (3) excellent behavior (3), and high effort (2).

One aspect of the observational design is the selection of the item types or method that will define the response format used. Multiple-choice items define one type of response format that can be used as part of observational design for measuring educational achievement. Items can be viewed generically as ranging from selected response or multiple-choice formats (pick the

Table 4.2   Guttman Mapping Sentence for Teacher Grading Practices

A teacher considers	Student characteristics			
	Ability	*Achievement*	*Behavior*	*Effort*
	1. Low	1. Low	1. Inappropriate	1. Low
	2. Average	2. Average	2. Average	2. High
	3. High	3. High	3. Excellent	
and				
	Grade			
	1. A			
then assigns a	2. B			
	3. C			
	4. D			
	5. F			

Adapted from Randall, J. & Engelhard G., 2009. Examining teacher grades using Rasch measurement theory. *Journal of Educational Measurement, 46*(1) 1–18.

Table 4.3   Sample Items

Facet →	*Ability*	*Achievement*	*Behavior*	*Effort*
Struct Item (*Structuple*)	*High (3)*	*High (3)*	*Excellent (3)*	*High (2)*
	Jonathan is a student with high ability, based on intelligence tests administered by the school. His behavior in class is always excellent. He rarely talks out of turn and has great manners. He tries hard and, based on project, test and quiz scores, you know that he has mastered 89% of the course objectives			
Struct Item (*Structuple*)	*Average (2)*	*High (3)*	*Low (1)*	*Low (1)*
	Glenda is a student with average ability, based on intelligence tests administered by the school. Her behavior is completely inappropriate. She talks out of turn often in class and is often disobedient. She does not work very hard, but based on project, test and quiz scores, you know that she has mastered 89% of the course objectives.			
Struct Item (*Structuple*)	*Average (2)*	*Low (1)*	*High (3)*	*High (2)*
	Willie is a student with average ability, based on intelligence tests administered by the school. His behavior in class is always excellent. He rarely talks out of turn and has great manners. He works very hard, but based on project, test and quiz scores, you know that he has mastered 69% of the course objectives.			
Struct Item (*Structuple*)	*Low (1)*	*Average (2)*	*Low (1)*	*Low (1)*
	Donna is a student with low ability, based on intelligence tests administered by the school. Her behavior is completely inappropriate. She talks out of turn often in class and is often disobedient. She does not work hard, and based on project, test and quiz scores, you know that she has mastered 89% of the course objectives.			

Adapted from Randall, J. & Engelhard G., 2009. Examining teacher grades using Rasch measurement theory. *Journal of Educational Measurement, 46*(1) 1–18.

right answer from among a set of distracters connected to an item stem—for example, a reading passage with 4 to 5 items designed to examine a student's reading achievement) to essay and other performance-based items. Constructed-responses involve students responding to a task or task shell. Examples would include the writing prompts used to measurement writing achievement.

Recent work on evidence-centered design is also becoming a popular method for designing educational assessments (Mislevy & Haertel, 2006). Evidence-centered design places assessments squarely in the realm of evidentiary arguments that can be used to guide the test validation process (Kane, 2006). Future work on developing observational designs should be carefully considered in the area of evidence-centered design.

In summary, observational designs guide the researcher in the construction of a plan for collecting systematic responses or observations from persons that inform inferences regarding where the person is located on the latent variable. In creating an observational design within the context of educational assessment, the researcher should consider the following questions:

Content: What do we want students to know?
Level: What do we want students to do with this knowledge?
Process: What do we want students to do next?

Wilson (2005) provides a generic description for these first two questions that he labels construct components (content) and distributional components (levels). The third question reflects a concern with formative assessments that provide diagnostic and feedback information to both students and teachers regarding the next aspect of an instructional sequence. The observational design specifies the substantive definition of the content, as well as the conditions used to collect the information on the observations. The researcher constructing a measure selects a finite set of items or structured observations that are designed to define and represent the latent variable. Wilson (2005) should be consulted for additional information regarding aspects of observational designs.

The major question undergirding this section is: What is the plan for collecting structured observations or responses from persons in order to define the latent variable? The important sub-questions are (a) What are the construct components (content—knowing) of the latent variable?, (b) What are the distributional components (levels/categories—doing)?, (c) What should students learn next in their sequence of instruction, and (d) What item formats are being used?

3. Scoring Rules: How Do We Categorize the Systematic Observations, and then Assign Scores to the Categories To Be Used as Indicators of the Latent Variable?

Scoring rules provide a detailed description of how to map categories of observations into scores. These scoring rules define the process used to categorize observations, and then they are used to score them as indicators of the construct (Wilson, 2005). The scoring rules address how to categorize person responses to situations defined by the observational design or items described in the previous section. In the case of multiple-choice items, the scoring rules are reflected in the answer key that identifies the choice or option presented to the person that has been identified a priori as the right answer (or best answer). Scoring rules can include dichotomous and polytomous rules to create rating scales and partial-credit scales. In essence, scoring rules are the strategies for coding responses from a domain or outcome space onto the variable map or line that represents the latent variable.

Returning to Figure 4.3, there are several possible scoring rules that might be used. For example, the researcher might define the latent variable as size with the smallest stars in Category 1 and the largest stars in Category 3. The research might simply assign the scores of 0, 1, and 2 to these three categories:

Category:	Category 1	Category 2	Category 3
Observations:	f, g, n, k,	d, h, j, l, m, o	b, c, e, p
Scores:	0	1	2

Or in the second example, the researcher might decide to map by shading with a null category with only two scoring categories

Category:	Category 1	Category 2	Category 3
Observations:	a, i	b, c, d, e, h, j, l, m, o	f, k, n, p
Scores:	0	0	1

The scoring rules for multiple-choice items with four distracters (one correct answer indicated by an asterisk) can be viewed as follows:

Distractors	Scores	Note
a	0	Wrong
b*	1	Correct answer
c	0	Wrong
d	0	Wrong

As another example of a scoring rule, an AP English Literature and Composition Exam asks students to respond to three constructed-response questions (Engelhard & Myford, 2003), and the third constructed-response question was scored with the rubric shown in Figure 4.5. As was the case with categorizing stars, the scoring rule for the observations (essays in this case) suggests ways to categorize observations on the latent variable from low to high on a continuum.

Ideally, the scoring rules yield well-defined, finite, and exhaustive categories. These categories are ordered and context-specific. The categories and scoring rules define the framework that was used to assign numbers to the categories, and reflect amount or degree of the latent variable on the underlying continuum. The important questions are how to categorize observations, and then how to develop a set of scoring rules to use these categories as indicators where persons and items are located on the latent variable or construct.

The key question in this section is: How are observations or responses categorized to represent person locations and levels on the latent variable? The sub-questions are (a) What are the definitions for categories or performance levels of persons that are measured? and (b) How are categories scored (scoring scheme)?

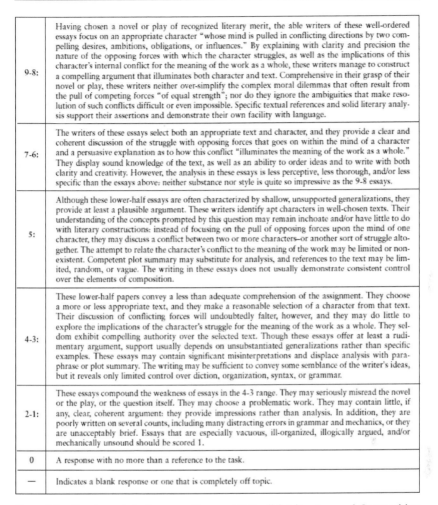

9-8:	Having chosen a novel or play of recognized literary merit, the able writers of these well-ordered essays focus on an appropriate character "whose mind is pulled in conflicting directions by two compelling desires, ambitions, obligations, or influences." By explaining with clarity and precision the nature of the opposing forces with which the character struggles, as well as the implications of this character's internal conflict for the meaning of the work as a whole, these writers manage to construct a compelling argument that illuminates both character and text. Comprehensive in their grasp of their novel or play, these writers neither over-simplify the complex moral dilemmas that often result from the pull of competing forces "of equal strength"; nor do they ignore the ambiguities that make resolution of such conflicts difficult or even impossible. Specific textual references and solid literary analysis support their assertions and demonstrate their own facility with language.
7-6:	The writers of these essays select both an appropriate text and character, and they provide a clear and coherent discussion of the struggle with opposing forces that goes on within the mind of a character and a persuasive explanation as to how this conflict "illuminates the meaning of the work as a whole." They display sound knowledge of the text, as well as an ability to order ideas and to write with both clarity and creativity. However, the analysis in these essays is less perceptive, less thorough, and/or less specific than the essays above: neither substance nor style is quite so impressive as the 9-8 essays.
5:	Although these lower-half essays are often characterized by shallow, unsupported generalizations, they provide at least a plausible argument. These writers identify apt characters in well-chosen texts. Their understanding of the concepts prompted by this question may remain inchoate and/or have little to do with literary constructions: instead of focusing on the pull of opposing forces upon the mind of one character, they may discuss a conflict between two or more characters–or another sort of struggle altogether. The attempt to relate the character's conflict to the meaning of the work may be limited or non-existent. Competent plot summary may substitute for analysis, and references to the text may be limited, random, or vague. The writing in these essays does not usually demonstrate consistent control over the elements of composition.
4-3:	These lower-half papers convey a less than adequate comprehension of the assignment. They choose a more or less appropriate text, and they make a reasonable selection of a character from that text. Their discussion of conflicting forces will undoubtedly falter, however, and they may do little to explore the implications of the character's struggle for the meaning of the work as a whole. They seldom exhibit compelling authority over the selected text. Though these essays offer at least a rudimentary argument, support usually depends on unsubstantiated generalizations rather than specific examples. These essays may contain significant misinterpretations and displace analysis with paraphrase or plot summary. The writing may be sufficient to convey some semblance of the writer's ideas, but it reveals only limited control over diction, organization, syntax, or grammar.
2-1:	These essays compound the weakness of essays in the 4-3 range. They may seriously misread the novel or the play, or the question itself. They may choose a problematic work. They may contain little, if any, clear, coherent argument: they provide impressions rather than analysis. In addition, they are poorly written on several counts, including many distracting errors in grammar and mechanics, or they are unacceptably brief. Essays that are especially vacuous, ill-organized, illogically argued, and/or mechanically unsound should be scored 1.
0	A response with no more than a reference to the task.
—	Indicates a blank response or one that is completely off topic.

Figure 4.5   Scoring rubric for a question on AP English Literature and Composition Exam.

4. Rasch Measurement Model: How Are Person and Item Responses or Observations Mapped onto the Latent Variable?

The fourth building block is the measurement model. In this book, the Rasch model is the measurement model. There are other item response theory models that can be used, but these models do not meet the requirements of invariant measurement as defined in this book. Van der Linden and Hambleton (1997) should be consulted for an authoritative description of the major models in item response theory. Crocker and Algina (1986) provide an overview of other test theory models including classical test theory, generalizability theory, and factor analysis. The Rasch model is used exclusively in this book because it is the only model that meets the requirements of invariant measurement. The Rasch model provides the rules for mapping both persons and items onto the latent variable. It provides the connections between scores, responses and the latent variable. Item locations are determined by the calibration of item responses using Rasch measurement. It also provides the link for placing persons on the same scale. The dichotomous Rasch model allows the calibration of items and the measurement of persons on a latent variable. The Rasch measurement model describes a theoretical framework for relating the scored responses from persons based on the observational design to locations on the latent variable that defines the variable map.

The measurement model relates scores to the latent variable as a function of location of persons and items on the scale or underlying continuum. In a sense, a measurement model is a psychometric model that reflects the application of a statistical model to a data set designed to address issues related to measurement. The Rasch measurement model is used to estimate the probability of dichotomous item responses as a logistic function of the difference between item and person locations on the latent variable. The Rasch model for the dichotomous case can be written as follows for a correct response (x = 1)

$$P_{ni1} = Pr\,(x_{ni} = 1|\theta_n,\delta_i) = exp(\theta_n - \delta_i)/\,[1 + exp(\theta_n - \delta_i)],$$

and for an incorrect response (x = 0)

$$P_{ni0} = Pr\,(x_{ni} = 0|\theta_n,\delta_i) = 1\,/\,[1 + exp(\theta_n - \delta_i)]$$

where x_{ni} is the observed response from person n on item i (0 = incorrect, 1= right), θ_n is the location of person n on the latent variable, and δ_i is the location (difficulty) of item i on the same scale. Once estimates of θ_n and δ_i are available, then the probability of each item response and item response pattern can be calculated based on the Rasch model. Additional details regarding the derivation of this model, the estimation of the person and item parameters, and the role of requirements of invariant measurement in the development of Rasch models are presented in other chapters. In terms of this building block, the important point is that the Rasch model provides the statistical and psychometric machinery for connecting responses with item and person locations in terms of logistic models that can be used to create variable maps.

This section addresses the important question regarding: How are person and item responses or observations mapped onto the latent variable? Related to this question is a concern with evidence regarding the following questions: Do the locations of persons and items match the hypothesized order proposed by the researcher in the hypothesized variable map? It is also important to consider issues related to quality control related to this question: How well do the persons and items fit the requirements of the Rasch model?

In summary, the building blocks described in the previous four sections provide a framework that supports the ultimate goal of creating a variable map. The variable map provides a visual display of the latent variable with locations of both persons and items. It also provides a coherent, substantive definition of content and level of observations mapped onto an underlying continuum with both persons and items ordered from less to more. As pointed out earlier, variable maps have also been called construct maps, item maps, curriculum maps, and Wright maps, named in honor of Ben Wright (Wilson, 2005). The key question is how to collect observations with the aim of gathering evidence and drawing inferences regarding the location of both persons and items on the latent variable or construct being measured. In the next two sections, two examples are provided to illustrate how these building blocks can be applied to build useful measures.

Applications

The next two sections provide applications of the four building blocks to the assessment of the home environments of preschool children and the assessment of the knowledge of nurses regarding the safe administration of medications.

I. Learning Stimulation in the Home Environments of Preschool Children

This section briefly illustrates the application of the building blocks to the problem of measuring the learning stimulation available in the home environments of preschool children. The data presented in this section are based on Monsaas and Engelhard (1996), and the actual data were presented in Chapter 1. Table 4.4 presents the underlying questions for the building blocks, and the guiding answers that undergird this study. Learning stimulation is the latent variable, and the purpose of this study is to measure the opportunities for learning stimulation provided in the home environments of preschool children. The learning stimulation scale is composed of 11 items that are checked by observers as not present or present. The judgments regarding presence of learning opportunities in the home environment were made by teachers visiting families in their homes. It is assumed that the more activities and objects available in the home, the higher the level of learning stimulation in the home environment. A dichotomous Rasch model was used to connect the responses (judgments of absence or presence of the 11 items on the scale to inferences regarding the location of persons and items on the learning stimulation continuum.

Figure 4.6 is the variable map for the learning stimulation scale, and it presents the empirical variable map obtained from the Facets computer program. The Facets computer program (Linacre, 2007) is used for all of the examples in this book. This version of the variable map can be compared with the hypothesized representation of the construct in Figure 1.2 of Chapter 1. The first column is the logit scale. Column 2 maps the location of each home

Table 4.4   Building Blocks for Creating Variable Map for Learning Stimulation Scale (LS Scale)

Building Blocks	Questions	Answers	Learning Stimulation (LS) Scale
Latent variable	What is the latent variable being measured?	Learning Stimulation	The purpose of the LS scale is to measure the degree of learning stimulation in the home environment of preschool children.
Observational design	What is the plan for collecting structured responses or observations from persons?	Items: List of activities available in the home environment	Dichotomous ratings obtained from teachers visiting the homes of preschool children
Scoring rules	How are responses or observations categorized to represent person levels on the latent variable?	Objects and activities scored not present (x=0) or present (x=1)	Activities and objects checked as present indicate a higher level of learning stimulation in the home environment (0=not present, 1=present)
Measurement model	How are person and item responses or observations mapped onto the latent variable?	Rasch model	Dichotomous Rasch model

environment on this scale with Persons 1, 9, and 28 living in home environments that have a high level of learning stimulation, while Persons 19, 33, and 36 live in home environments with lower levels of stimulation for learning. The last column operationally defines the actual items or observations that were used to draw inferences regarding where a person's home environment falls on this scale. It is relatively easy to find toys and shape learning in most of the home environments. It was harder to find magazines, music players, newspapers, and puzzles in these home environments. Details of how to construct this particular variable map are presented later.

2. Assessment in the Health Sciences: The Five Rights of Safe Administration of Medications

This section briefly describes the Safe Administration of Medication (SAM) Scale developed by Debra Ryan in her dissertation at Emory University. The SAM scale was designed to explore the medication errors of nurses. This is a significant concern in today's healthcare environment. Numerous studies have focused on adverse drug events and the significance of these events on patient

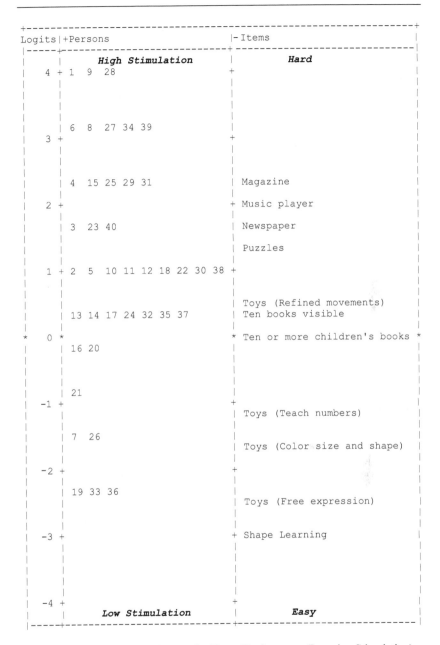

```
+----------------------------------------------------------------+
|                                                                |
Logits|+Persons                         |-Items                    |
|-----+---------------------------------+--------------------------|
|     |        High Stimulation         |          Hard            |
|   4 + 1  9  28                         +                          |
|     |                                  |                          |
|     |                                  |                          |
|     |                                  |                          |
|     | 6  8  27 34 39                   |                          |
|   3 +                                  +                          |
|     |                                  |                          |
|     |                                  |                          |
|     | 4  15 25 29 31                   | Magazine                 |
|     |                                  |                          |
|   2 +                                  + Music player             |
|     |                                  |                          |
|     | 3  23 40                         | Newspaper                |
|     |                                  |                          |
|     |                                  | Puzzles                  |
|     |                                  |                          |
|   1 + 2  5  10 11 12 18 22 30 38       +                          |
|     |                                  |                          |
|     |                                  |                          |
|     |                                  | Toys (Refined movements) |
|     | 13 14 17 24 32 35 37             | Ten books visible        |
|     |                                  |                          |
*  0 *                                   * Ten or more children's books *
|     | 16 20                            |                          |
|     |                                  |                          |
|     |                                  |                          |
|     | 21                               |                          |
|  -1 +                                  +                          |
|     |                                  | Toys (Teach numbers)     |
|     |                                  |                          |
|     | 7  26                            |                          |
|     |                                  | Toys (Color size and shape) |
|     |                                  |                          |
|  -2 +                                  +                          |
|     |                                  |                          |
|     | 19 33 36                         |                          |
|     |                                  | Toys (Free expression)   |
|     |                                  |                          |
|     |                                  |                          |
|  -3 +                                  + Shape Learning           |
|     |                                  |                          |
|     |                                  |                          |
|     |                                  |                          |
|     |                                  |                          |
|  -4 +                                  +                          |
|     |        Low Stimulation          |          Easy            |
|-----+---------------------------------+--------------------------|
```

Figure 4.6   Empirical Variable Map for Home Environment (Learning Stimulation).

safety (Ryan, 2007). Patient safety is dependent on nurses who consistently demonstrate behaviors fundamental to safe administration of medications. Student nurses who are unable to demonstrate these behaviors need additional learning opportunities to develop skills consistent with safe practices.

The SAM Scale was designed to objectively measure the proficiency of student nurses to identify medication errors. The specific areas measured relate to the responsibility of nurses in ensuring the five rights of safe administration of medications. These five rights are right patient, right drug, right dose, right time, and right route; opportunities for errors occur each time a medication is administered by a nurse. The SAM Scale is a paper and pencil instrument that provides a series of five clinical cases describing hypothetical patients and 14 vignettes describing nurse behaviors regarding the administration of a drug. Each case provides patient information, chief complaint, history and physical diagnosis, physician orders, and medication orders. The vignettes include a description of various errors made by hypothetical nurses. The task for the student nurses is to correctly identify the errors made in the administration of the drug based on information provided in the case studies and vignettes.

Table 4.5 presents the underlying questions for the building blocks, and the guiding answers that undergird this study. Proficiency of student nurses in identifying principles of safe administration of medications is the latent variable. The SAM scale is composed of five clinical case studies with 14 vignettes. This yields 70 possible scoring opportunities for incorrectly or correctly identifying errors in administering medications. It is assumed that the more errors identified by student nurses, the higher their level of proficiency in the safe administration of medications. A dichotomous Rasch model was used to connect the responses (incorrect or correct identification of medication errors) to inference regarding the location of persons and items on the proficiency continuum.

The guiding variable map for the SAM Scale is shown in Figure 4.7. The student nurses are measured on a continuum that ranges from decreasing to increasing proficiency in the safe administration of medications. The performance items based on the five rights of safe administration of medications are hypothesized to range from easy items that ask the nurse to confirm that the right patient is receiving the drug to more difficult items that represent the confirmation of proper dosage for the patient.

Discussion and Summary

The purpose of this chapter was to briefly describe the basic building blocks that are necessary for constructing variable maps. Four building blocks for researcher-constructed measures were described in this chapter; specifically, these include the latent variable, the observational design (items), the scoring rules (performance levels), and the Rasch measurement model. These building blocks were shown to form a conceptually sound basis to guide researchers

Table 4.5 Building Blocks for Creating Variable Map for Safe Administration of Medication Scale (SAM Scale)

Building Blocks	Questions	Answers	Safe Administration of Medications (SAM Scale)
Latent variable	What is the latent variable being measured?	Proficiency of student nurses in identifying principles of safe administration of medications	The purpose of the SAM Scale is to objectively measure student the proficiency of student nurses to identify medication errors.
Observational design	What is the plan for collecting structured responses or observations from persons?	Five clinical case studies with 14 vignettes describing nurse behaviors	Paper and pencil instrument that provides a series of five clinical cases describing hypothetical patients. Each case provides patient information, chief complaint, history & physical, diagnosis, physician orders and medication orders.
Scoring rules	How are responses or observations categorized to represent person levels on the latent variable?	Vignettes are scored x=0 (error not detected) , x=1 (error detected)	Student nurse responses are scored dichotomously based on whether they detect the medication error.
Measurement model	How are person and item responses or observations mapped onto the latent variable?	Rasch model	Dichotomous Rasch model

in their development of psychometrically defensible measures. The interested reader is encouraged to read Wilson (2005) for additional details regarding his approach to constructing measures based on an item response modeling approach.

In summary, the construction of an instrument to measure a latent variable or construct that is of theoretical interest and substantive utility involves a number of steps. It is important to specify the variable map in detail. Ideally, this should include the motivation for creating the instrument and the intended purposes or uses of the information obtained from persons. It is also important to specify an observational design for defining, generating, and categorizing observations or responses that have hypothesized locations on the variable map used to represent the latent variable. Closely related to the observational

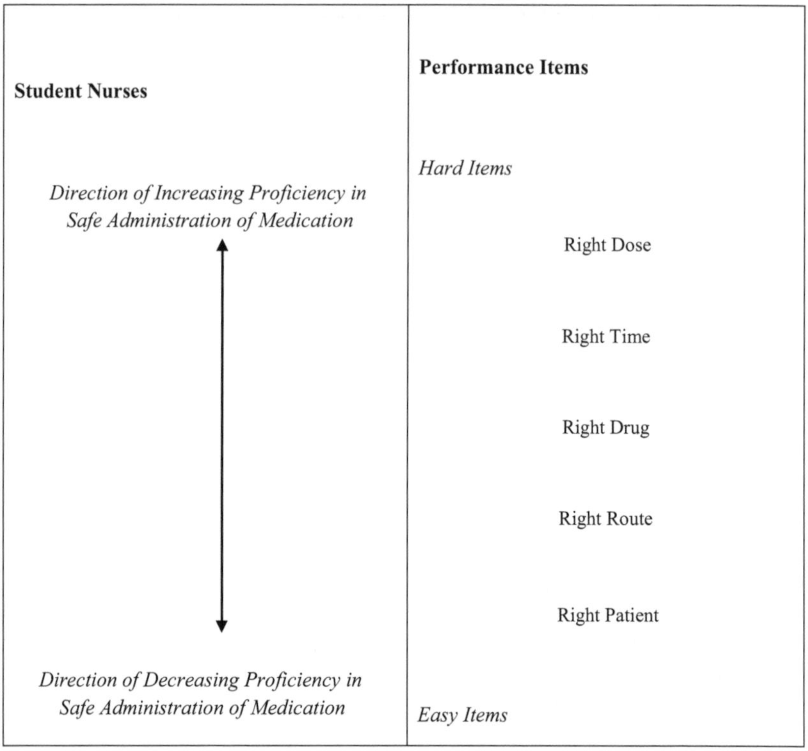

Student Nurses	Performance Items
Direction of Increasing Proficiency in Safe Administration of Medication ↑ │ │ │ │ ↓	*Hard Items* Right Dose Right Time Right Drug Right Route Right Patient
Direction of Decreasing Proficiency in Safe Administration of Medication	*Easy Items*

Adapted from Ryan, D.D. Measurement of student nurse performance in the safe
administration of medication. Unpublished doctoral dissertation, Emory University. 2007.

Figure 4.7   Variable map for Safe Administration of Medication Scale.

design are considerations regarding the scoring rules that are used to assign
an order to the observations along the latent variable. Although these steps
or building blocks are described in a linear fashion, actual construction of an
instrument is a scientific process that involves several iterations with numerous feedback loops among the building blocks.

Chapter 5

An Historical and Comparative Perspective on Research Traditions in Measurement

The history of science is the history of measurement.

(Cattell, 1893, p. 316)

This chapter focuses on the history of ideas and theories about measurement in the social, behavioral, and health sciences.[1] Historical, philosophical, and comparative perspectives on invariant measurement are presented using selected measurement theories and theorists to illustrate the key themes. This chapter should be considered an initial step towards the development of a history of ideas about social science measurement in general and invariant measurement in particular. I recognize that contextual factors, such as the social, cultural, and political issues, are important in the history of assessment, but a thorough discussion of these contextual issues is not the major focus of this chapter. Porter (1986, 1995), Dubois (1970), and Linden and Linden (1968) provide useful starting points for readers interested in the broader social, cultural and political context of assessment in the human sciences.

This chapter is organized around the view that the dominant measurement theories developed and used during the 20th century can be meaningfully classified into two major research traditions or paradigms that I call the test-score and scaling tradition. The methodology used in this chapter is based on a deep and detailed reading of the published work of selected measurement theorists.

---

1   On a personal note, much of the work in this chapter was started in a graduate seminar with Professor Ben Wright at the University of Chicago. In this seminar, I focused on the historical adumbrations of the ideas undergirding invariant measurement. In a series of articles and chapters over the past 25 or so years, I have explored the historical context of this quest for invariant measurement within the work of several key measurement theorists including Thorndike, Thurstone, Lazarsfeld, Mokken, Rasch, Guttman, and others. One of my major findings was that a number of perennial problems in measurement theory can be productively viewed through the theoretical lens of invariant measurement. This chapter is based on my program of historical and philosophical research, and also includes analyses of several major measurement theorists not included in my earlier work.

In essence, the published writing of each measurement theorist becomes the "data" that support my inferences regarding various views of measurement in the human sciences. The supporting data include not only text, but the equations, tables, figures, and other visual displays created by these measurement theorists. I have tried to avoid the historical error of presentism (viewing the past through the lens of the present), and I recognize that quotations when taken out of context can have their meaning distorted. I urge the motivated reader to view this chapter as an introduction to key measurement ideas, and to seek out and read the original work of the measurement theorists included in this chapter. It is well worth the effort. It should also be stressed that this chapter does not draw a distinction between history and philosophy of measurement. As pointed out by Laudan (1977, 1990) the gap between dealing with "facts" as historical components versus "values" as philosophical components in science are quite artificial, and they do not reflect how science is actually conducted. Therefore, this chapter is both historical and philosophical in nature with the inclusion of a guided view of what assessment can and should be within the larger framework of invariant measurement in the social, behavioral, and health sciences.

There were numerous theories of measurement proposed and used during the 20th century. It is argued that these theories can be productively viewed as being grouped under two general research traditions. This is not intended to ignore the nuances of each particular measurement theory, but to provide a broader conceptual framework that can be used to highlight concepts and issues related to the quest for invariant measurement in the social, behavioral, and health sciences. I have tried to capture the ebb and flow of various traditions as reflected in particular measurement theories that best represent key ideas and issues. No claim is made that an exhaustive description of all measurement theories is provided.

In the first section of this chapter, I describe the general view of measurement theories used in this book. Next, the concept of research traditions is introduced as an organizing principle for viewing the measurement theories. The following section proposes two broad categories (test-score and scaling traditions) as an organizing framework for viewing measurement theories. Next, specific measurement theories within the test-score tradition are described. The specific measurement theories included in the test-score tradition are classical test theory, generalizability theory, factor analysis, and structural equation models. Next, the major measurement theories that can be classified under the scaling tradition are presented. Illustrative theories from the scaling tradition are represented by the measurement research with theories rooted in psychophysics, absolute scaling, item response theory and non-parametric item response theory.

What Are Measurement Theories?

Measurement theories can be defined in a variety of ways. In this book, the basic definition of measurement theory is based on the work of Messick (1983):

> Theories of measurement broadly conceived may be viewed as loosely integrated conceptual frameworks within which are embedded rigorously formulated statistical models of estimation and inference about the properties of measurements and scores. (p. 498)

There are several aspects of this definition that should be highlighted. First of all, Messick (1983) is defining measurement as a conceptual framework or set of ideas about measurement processes. This underlying theory defines the basic requirements and aspects of measurement. For example, one of the most commonly cited definitions of measurement was proposed by Stevens (1946): "measurement, in its broadest sense, is defined as the assignment of numerals to objects or events according to rules" (p. 677). This definition begs the question of what "rules" are being used. As pointed out by Ellis (1968), it is important to go further:

> The mere possession of a rule, therefore, does not ensure that we have a scale of measurement ... we have a scale of measurement only if the following conditions are satisfied:
> (a) we have a rule for making numerical assignments;
> (b) this rule is *determinative* in the sense that, provided sufficient care is exercised the same numeral (or ranges of numerals) would always be assigned to the same things under the same conditions;
> (c) the rule is non-degenerate in the sense that it allows for the possibility of assigning different numerals (or ranges of numerals) to different things, or to the same thing under different conditions. (p. 41)

The determinative nature of the conditions proposed by Ellis (1968) suggests that measurement requirements defined as rules should be specified a priori. It is argued that ideal-type scales proposed by Guttman (1950), Rasch (1960/1980), and Mokken (1971) can meet the requirements for invariant measurement. In essence, measurement theories provide the rules that specify the requirements for measurement, and the guidelines for the development of empirical measures based on these requirements. Requirements undergird the rules, and they provide the conceptual framework for each particular measurement theory.

Messick (1983) suggests that theoretical frameworks are embedded within a particular model. This is a source of confusion for many measurement practitioners who tend to confuse the underlying statistical model with the broader conceptual framework that defines various measurement theories. For example, many of the aspects of classical test theory are grounded in correlational methods developed concurrently within this statistical framework. As another example, generalizability theory and other extensions of classical test theory are based on statistical advances in agricultural experimentation, such as the design of experiments that led to analysis of variance models. More recently, advances in item response theory are based on fundamental developments and advances in the analysis of categorical and ordinal data in the statistics literature. A major point here is that the statistical machinery is part of the model, but a full consideration of the measurement theory requires a consideration of the broader conceptual and theoretical framework that contextualizes the statistical aspects of the model. Both the conceptual framework and the statistical aspects of the model combine to provide the basis for drawing inferences from scores. As pointed out by Wright (1997), all measurements are inferences, and the trick is to go from what we have—observations from person responses to a set of task or test items—to useful measurement regarding the location of both persons and items on an underlying latent variable or construct. These inferences regarding measurements form the input to our decisions for theory, practice and policy in the social, behavioral, and health sciences.

The underlying motivation for studying the conceptual frameworks, statistical models, and inferences from our measurement theories has been succinctly stated by Lazarsfeld (1966):

> Problems of concept formation, of meaning, and of measurement necessarily fuse into each other ... measurement, classification and concept formation in the behavioral sciences exhibit special difficulties. They can be met by a variety of procedures, and only a careful analysis of the procedure and its relation to alternative solutions can clarify the problem itself, which the procedure attempts to solve. (p. 144).

In essence, Messick (1983) and Lazarsfeld (1966) stress that measurement theories are of key importance because they

*   define the aspects of quantification that are defined as problematic,
*   determine the statistical models and appropriate methods used to solve these problems,
*   determine the impact of our research in the social, behavioral, and health sciences,
*   frame the substantive conclusions and inferences that we draw, and ultimately
*   delineate and limit the policies and practices derived from our research work in the social, behavioral, and health sciences.

In the next section, the concept of research traditions is introduced and used to structure the discussion of the various measurement theories.

What Are Research Traditions?

Philosophy of science without history of science is empty; history of science without philosophy of science is blind.

(Lakatos, 1971, p. 91)

What we need, if our appraisals of [alternative theories] are to be at all reliable, is serious historical scholarship devoted to the various research traditions in a given field of inquiry.

(Laudan, 1977, p. 194)

Laudan (1977) proposed the concept of a research tradition. Research traditions are similar to paradigms (Kuhn, 1970), research programs (Lakatos, 1978), and disciplines (Cronbach, 1957, 1975). It is helpful to organize our thinking about the history of measurement theory around the concept of research traditions. Research traditions can provide a useful set of categories for examining theories of measurement. According to Laudan (1977),

we have thus far characterized research traditions as rather ambitious and grandiose entities, replete with ontologies and methodologies. There is no doubt in my mind that many of the best known research traditions in science possess both these characteristics. But there also seem to be traditions and schools in science which, although lacking one or the other (or in some cases both), have nonetheless had a genuine intellectual coherence about them. For instance, the tradition of psychometrics in the early twentieth century seems to have held together by little more than the conviction that mental phenomena could be mathematically represented. (p. 105)

A research tradition has the following characteristics: (a) it defines the aspects of quantification which are viewed as problematic, (b) it defines the methods which can be used to address these problems, and finally, (c) through the definition of measurement problems and methods, a research tradition has a significant impact on how social science research is conducted (Laudan, 1977). Different research traditions imply different assumptions and requirements, as well as different ways of viewing research and the conceptualization of assessment.

This chapter suggests that two major research traditions have dominated measurement in the 20th century: the test-score tradition and the scaling tradition. This distinction goes back to Torgerson (1961) who organized his chapter on assessment in the first annual review of psychology under the title: test theory and scaling, as well as the earlier work of Mosier (1940, 1941). The next section presents and describes these two major research traditions.

What Are the Two Major Research Traditions in Measurement?

There are two dominant research traditions in measurement theory: the test-score tradition and the scaling tradition. As its label implies, the test-score tradition focuses on test scores with a primary concern with measurement error, and the decomposition of an observed test score into several components including a true score with various error components. This tradition has its roots in the psychometric work of Spearman (1904a), and continues in the work on classical test theory (Traub, 1997), generalizability theory (Brennan, 1997; Cronbach, Gleser, Nanda, and Rajaratnam, 1972), factor analysis (Cudeck & MacCallum, 2007) and structural equation models (Joreskog, 2007).

Scaling theory is the second dominant research tradition in measurement theory. Scaling theory has its roots in 19th-century psychophysics, and it has continued to the present through various forms of item response theory (Bock, 1997; Rasch, 1960/1980; van der Linden & Hambleton, 1997). The focus of the scaling theory tradition is on the creation of a variable map that represents the location of both items and persons onto a latent variable scale that represents a construct. In some cases, the scaling models focus primarily on mapping persons, and in other models the focus is on mapping both persons and items on the variable map. It should be stressed that the five requirements of invariant measurement (item-invariant measurement of persons, non-crossing person response functions, person-invariant calibration of items, non-crossing item response functions, and variable maps) must be met to achieve the goal of simultaneously mapping both persons and items on the same construct or latent variable scale.

Table 5.1 provides an overview of the classification of measurement theories based on the test-score and scaling traditions discussed in this chapter.

Test-Score Tradition

Classical test theory (CTT) was developed in the early 20th century, and it represents the genesis of the test-score tradition. CTT is based on three key ideas: measurements have errors, these errors can be modeled as a random variable, and correlation coefficients can be corrected for these measurement errors to produce so called disattenuated correlations. The key figure in the development of CTT is Spearman (1904a) who proposed a method for correcting correlations coefficients to account for measurement errors—his correction for attenuation. Traub (1997) identified five milestones in the development of classical test theory: Spearman's correction for attenuation, the Spearman-Brown formula, the index of reliability, the Kuder-Richardson formulas, and lower bounds to reliability. See Traub (1997) for a description of each of these milestones.

Table 5.1   Two Research Traditions for Classifying Measurement Theories

Test-Score Tradition	*Scaling Tradition*
Key models:	Key models:
1. Classical test theory (CTT)	1. Psychophysical models (PM)
2. Generalizability theory (GT)	2. Absolute Scaling (AS)
3. Factor analysis (FA)	3. Item Response Theory (IRT)
4. Structural equation modeling (SEM)	4. Non-Parametric Item Response Theory (NIRT)
Essential features:	Essential features:
Test-score focus	Item-person response focus
Linear models	Non-linear models
Focus on test scores and the estimation of error components	Focus on modeling the responses of persons to items
Key theorists and models:	Key theorists and models:
Spearman (CTT)	Thorndike (PM)
Kuder and Richardson (CTT)	Thurstone (AS)
Cronbach and his colleagues (GT)	Birnbaum (IRT)
Spearman (FA)	Rasch (IRT)
Thurstone (FA)	Guttman (NIRT)
Joreskog (SEM)	Lazarsfeld (NIRT)
	Mokken (NIRT)
Theory into practice:	Theory into practice:
Brennan (GT)	Lord (IRT: Birnbaum)
Joreskog (SEM)	Wright (IRT: Rasch)

The two key references for classical test theory are Gulliksen (1950) and Lord and Novick (1968). In the next section, several theories within the test-score tradition are described. The test-score tradition tends to focus on the "variant" aspects of measurement models with a focus on the quantification of sources of error variance. This stands in contrast to theories within the scaling tradition that address many of the issues related to invariant measurement. The key measurement theorists used to represent the test-score tradition are Spearman (1904a), Cronbach, Rajaratnam, and Gleser (1963), Thurstone (1935), and Joreskog (1971). Each of these is briefly described in turn in the following sections.

I. The Founding of Classical Test Theory: Spearman

In the same year that Thorndike (1904) published his book on social science measurement, Spearman published a seminal article entitled: "General

Intelligence" objectively determined and measured (Spearman, 1904a). He also published several other articles that in combination laid the groundwork for classical test theory (Spearman, 1904b, 1907, 1910). Thorndike (1945) identified four major discoveries presented by Spearman (1904b). First of all, Spearman recognized that chance variations in measures always move correlations from their true values. Next, he proposed a procedure for adjusting the raw or observed correlations to correct for these chance variations or errors in measurement. Third, he developed a conceptual framework that would eventually lead to factor analysis and the work of Thurstone (1947). And finally, Spearman (1904a) introduced his views regarding general intelligence ("g") that would lead to decades of debate and controversy regarding whether human abilities should be viewed as being a function of a single underlying factor called "g" (general intelligence) or a function of multiple abilities (e.g., Thurstone's primary abilities).

In Spearman's work, it is clear that the core of classical test theory is based on the perspective that the observed test score for person n (X_n) is defined as the sum of two components: a true score (T_n) and a error score (E_n). This can be represented as follows:

$$X_n = T_n + E_n \qquad [1]$$

This decomposition of an observed score can be traced to earlier work by Carl Friedrich Gauss on the normal distribution. It should be stressed that this model for observed scores (X_n) does not directly relate to item characteristics. Instead, the focus is on the sum of item responses with no attempt to explicitly include item characteristics, such as item difficulty, in the model. Essentially, classical test theory uses the statistical methodology of correlation coefficients to solve psychometric issues related to the estimation of reliability coefficients.

Classical test theory is primarily concerned with the estimation of reliability coefficients. Two of the major milestones during the 20th century were the publication of the Kuder-Richardson formulas (Kuder & Richardson, 1937) and coefficient alpha (Cronbach, 1951). Later work in this classical test theory tradition stressed the role of reliability coefficients in estimating standard errors of measurement for interpretation of person scores. The major historical publications on classical test theory are by Spearman (1904b), Thurstone (1931), Gulliksen (1950), and Lord and Novick (1968).

2. Generalizability Theory: Cronbach and His Colleagues

An investigator asks about the precision or reliability of a measure because he wishes to generalize from the observation in hand to some class of observations to which it belongs. To ask about rater agreement is to ask how well we can generalize from a set of ratings to ratings by other raters. To ask about the reliability of an essay-examination grade is to ask how representative this is of a grade that might be given to the same paper by other markers, or of grades on other paper by the same subject.

(Cronbach et al., 1963, p. 144)

Classical test theory has been a dominant force in psychometrics with its influences continuing into the 21st century. As pointed out above, classical test theory focuses on measurement errors, and this concern with sources of error variance has been extended and elaborated upon within the context of generalizability theory. In essence, generalizability theory can be viewed as an application of mixed and random effects models (analysis of variance models) with multiple sources of random error. Generalizability (G) theory can be viewed as the merging of classical test theory and analysis of variance (Brennan, 1997). One of its first applications was within the context of rater-mediated assessments by Ebel (1951) on the reliability of ratings. Cronbach et al. (1963) and Brennan (1983) are key references regarding G theory. Interest in G theory has waxed and waned since its early development, but there has been a resurgence of interest in applications of G theory within the context of performance-based assessments in the human sciences. The model for generalizability theory is an extension of the one for classical test theory shown in Equation 1 with k additional error components added to the model. The underlying model is shown in Equation 2.

$$X_n = T_n + E_{n1} + E_{n2} + \ldots + E_{nk} \qquad [2]$$

In the G theory case, the observed test score for person n (X_n) is defined as the sum of a true score (T_n), and several error scores that may be due to items (E_{n1}), raters (E_{n2}), etc. Generalizability theory provides a framework for looking at item, rater and other facets of the assessment situation viewed as sources of error. The focus is on the analysis of sources of error variance within a multivariate structure. In essence, generalizability theory uses the statistical methodology underlying fixed and mixed effects ANOVA models to solve psychometric issues. Generalizability coefficients can be interpreted as the ratio of true score (corrected for various sources of error variance) to observed score variance.

Generalizability theory continues the tradition of classical test theory with a focus on summed item scores rather than the responses of persons to individual test items. It is not a scaling model, and it is sample dependent with a stress on estimating components of error variance in test scores. The major historical publications on generalizability theory are by Hoyt (1941) and Cronbach et al. (1972). Brennan (1983) provided the computer programs (GENOVA) that enhanced the practical utility of the generalizability theory.

3. Factor Analysis: Spearman and Thurstone

Spearman (1904a) laid the foundation for factor analysis. Much of the debate during the 20th century regarding human abilities within psychology was dominated by conflicting views regarding whether or not a single underlying latent variable or construct called intelligence ("g") accounts for the inter-correlations among tests of human performance. Spearman tended to support a unitary view of intelligence, while Thurstone (1938) identified multiple abilities underlying test performance. It is beyond the scope of this book to address the substantive aspects of this debate, but this issue provided the context within which the psychometric and statistical developments in factor analysis were conducted. See the edited volume by Cudeck and MacCallum (2007) for more details.

Factor analysis in its traditional form focuses on the reproduction of a matrix of correlations between a set of test scores with a smaller number of underlying factors or latent variables (Cudeck & MacCallum, 2007; McDonald, 1985; Spearman, 1927). The basic model can be represented as

$$X_n = \lambda_p T_n + E_n \qquad [3]$$

where the observed test score for person n (X_n) is defined as the sum of two components: a true score (T_n) weighted by a regression coefficient (λ_p) on test form p and a error score (E_n). Spearman's two-factor model defined the true score as a general ability factor, g, and the error score as a unique factor related to the particular form used.

In the 1930s, Thurstone (1935, 1936) introduced a multiple factor model as an alternative to Spearman's factor analysis model that had stressed a single underlying factor that Spearman called general ability. The multiple-factor model replaced this general factor (g) with a set of m common factors. Each person had a set of p scores from p tests, and the multiple-factor model can be written as follows:

$$X_{np} = \lambda_{n1} f_1 + \lambda_{n2} f_2 + \dots \lambda_{nm} f_p + E_{np} \qquad [4]$$

where the observed score of person n on form p is a weighted sum of m factors (f) with various weights (λ) for each factor

In practice, factor analysis models examine a set of p test forms. Factor analyses provide models for examining the inter-correlations among p test forms designed to measure the same true score. In matrix form, this can be written as

$$\Sigma_p = \hat{\Sigma}_p + E_p \qquad [5]$$

where Σ_p represents the observed correlation matrix among the p test scores, $\hat{\Sigma}_p$ represents the expected or reproduced correlation matrix based on estimation of a set of factors or latent variables, and E_p represents an error or residual matrix. It should be noted that we are one step removed from observed scores in this model. In fact, we are modeling a correlation or alternatively a variance-covariance matrix. The estimation and use of scores within this framework is very limited. In the practice of measurement in the human sciences, traditional factor analysis is typically used as a part of validity arguments, and then these analyses are set aside in the actual estimation of person scores. Early work on factor analysis focused on exploratory analyses. Later, confirmatory methods of factor analysis were introduced that provide a falsifiable framework for testing specific hypotheses that are particularly useful in measurement in the social, behavioral, and health sciences (Joreskog, 1969).

The close connection between classical test theory and factor analysis has been described by McDonald (1985). He illustrates how the classical estimators of reliability coefficients (e.g., test-retest reliability, equivalent forms reliability, and coefficient alpha), as well as generalizability coefficients can be viewed from a factor-analytic perspective. This adds support to the view that traditional factor analysis at its core is based on the test-score tradition. Recent advances in full information item factor analyses (Bock, Gibbons, & Muraki, 1988; Muraki & Engelhard, 1985) are not included in this section because the focus of these models is on item responses and multivariate item response theory rather than scores on several test forms. Item factor analysis models are more closely aligned with the scaling tradition, and they can be viewed as multidimensional item response models (Reckase, 2009).

Factor analysis is primarily used in current measurement practice as a part of the validity argument for the proposed interpretation of test scores. For example, the index to the latest edition of *Educational Measurement* (Brennan, 2006) includes only one entry for factor analysis, and this appears in the validity chapter. The validity section of the journal *Educational and Psychological Measurement* provides numerous examples of the use of factor analyses to validate inferences based on scores obtained from a variety of tests. Mulaik (1986) provides a history of the major developments in factor analysis. Yanai and Ichikawa (2007) provide a good summary of the basic issues in factor analysis.

4. Structural Equation Modeling: Joreskog

Structural equation modeling can be viewed as a combination of the factor analysis models with structural models (e.g., path analysis and regression models). One way to view structural equation models is to think of factor analysis as the method for identifying underlying latent variables or factors, and then these latent variables are used as the variables in the structural part of the structural equation. For example, a standard regression analysis would be conducted with the regression of an observed variable y on another observed variable x. A structural equation modeling approach might have multiple indicators of y and x, next a factor analysis would be conducted to identify the underlying latent variables for y' and x'. These factors or latent variables, y' and x', would then be included in the regression analysis.

Joreskog (1974, 2007) has worked extensively with statistical methods based on factor analysis and structural equation modeling to examine several psychometric issues. In essence, Joreskog suggested modeling covariance matrices directly. For example, his work on congeneric tests defines tests as congeneric if they measure the same latent variable except for measurement errors (Joreskog, 1971). Parallel tests and tau-equivalent tests based on the definitions of Lord and Novick (1968) are considered special cases of congeneric tests. The model of Equation 4 can be expanded to include several other matrices that can form the basis for very general analyses with structural equation models. It is beyond the scope of this book to delve into the possible ways of defining these aspects of the model, and Joreskog (2007) and Yuan and Bentler (2007) should be consulted for detailed descriptions of how to use structural equation models in the social, behavioral, and health sciences.

This section on test-traditions provides a general overview of selected models within this tradition. Due to their focus on error variances and measurement error, they provide less useful approaches to meet the requirements of invariant measurement as compared to the measurement models within the scaling tradition stressed in this book. Recent work by Milsap and Meredith (2007) has explored the problem of factorial invariance, and they have described how measurement invariance across groups can be examined within the framework of factor analysis and structural equation models.

The next section turns to the examination of selected measurement theories within the scaling tradition that holds promise for meeting the requirements of invariant measurement.

Scaling Tradition

The connections between the scaling tradition and measurement in the social, behavioral, and health sciences have their roots in 19th-century psychophysics. These connections between psychophysics and measurement have been recognized repeatedly, but they have not entered into the perspectives of most researchers within the human sciences. Psychophysics focuses on the scaling or calibration of stimuli (items and tasks), while measurement focuses on the scaling of responses from individuals. Psychophysics for example focused on how well people can distinguish variation in lifted weights and other aspects of sensory perceptions related to sight, hearing, smell, and taste. Key researchers in psychophysics were Fechner (1860) and Urban (1908).

Guilford (1936) in an early textbook also stressed the connection:

> The link between psychophysics and mental test is really a very direct and intimate one ... we see more clearly the common ground existing in

these two fields and a number of investigations have been instrumental in bridging the gap that has too long existed between them. It is one of the purposes of this volume to help point out the basic unity of the two fields and to assist in introducing one to the other. (pp.10–11)

A detailed treatment of this duality between psychophysics and mental tests appears in the work of Mosier (1940, 1941). According to Mosier (1940), the purpose of these two articles was:

> to reduce both disciplines [psychophysics and mental test theory] to their common postulational basis, in terms of their elements, definitions and assumptions, to deduce certain of the better known theorems of each field from these definitions and assumptions, and to show, since the two fields have a common basis of data and postulates, that it is possible by transposing certain terms, to restate the theorems of psychophysics for the mental test situation, and the theorems of mental test theory for the situations of psychophysics. (p. 355)

The scaling tradition has a number of distinct characteristics as represented by the measurement theories in this chapter. The single and most distinctive feature of the scaling tradition is development of a visual representation of the construct as a variable map.

Embretson (1996) has highlighted progress that has been made in the movement from the test-score tradition to the scaling tradition as represented by item response theory that she has called *the new rules of measurement*. Hambleton and Jones (1993) provide another useful comparison of measurement theories within a framework contrasting the test-score tradition (classical test theory) with the scaling tradition (item response theory).

The measurement theories within the scaling tradition can be further classified as parametric models (Thorndike, Thurstone, Birnbaum, and Rasch), and non-parametric models (Lazarsfeld, Guttman, and Mokken). Parametric models specify a priori the structure of the underlying operating characteristic functions, while nonparametric models do not limit the forms of the underlying operating characteristic functions. All of these models, parametric and non-parametric, are probabilistic in nature with the exception of Guttman scaling that is labeled a deterministic model. Probabilistic models hypothesize a stochastic relationship between the latent variables and person responses to a set of items. Also, Guttman and Rasch specified very clearly the a priori requirements of good measurement that qualifies each of them to be viewed as ideal-type models. Ideal-type models emphasize meeting the requirement of a measurement model in order to realize various desirable measurement characteristics, such as the requirements of invariant measurement highlighted in this book.

I. Psychophysics and the Beginning of the Scaling Tradition: Thorndike

Whatever exists, exists in some amount. To measure it is simply to know its vary-
ing amounts. Man sees no less beauty in flowers now than before the day of
quantitative botany.

(Thorndike, 1921, p. 379)

In 1904, E.L. Thorndike published his influential book entitled: *An Introduction to the Theory of Mental and Social Measurements*. According to Clifford (1984), Thorndike's book gained "a quick reputation as a tour de force: the first complete theoretical exposition and statistical handbook in the new area of social-science measurement" (p. 289). In this book, Thorndike clearly lays out the basic principles of measurement in the social sciences. His early work on social science measurement was strongly influenced by James McKeen Cattell who was his mentor at Columbia University (Clifford, 1984). Cattell (1893) had coined the term "mental test," and he was strongly grounded in 19th-century work in psychophysics by psychologists working in both Germany and England.

Thorndike had a deep appreciation for the creation and use of scales. Thorndike, with his colleagues and students, created numerous scales to measure several different latent variables, such as handwriting (1910), reading (1917), and writing (1916). These scales are conceptually equivalent to what would be recognized today as variable maps. Thorndike (1913) highlighted an early example of a "scale book' or variable map used by the Reverend George Fisher of Greenwich Hospital School and described by E. Chadwick in 1864. According Thorndike (1913):

> A book called the 'Scale-Book' has been established, which contains the numbers assigned to each degree of proficiency in the various subjects of examination: for instance, if it be required to determine the numerical equivalent corresponding to any specimen of 'writing,' a comparison is made with various standard specimens, which are arranged in this book in order of merit: the highest being represented by the number 1, and the lowest by 5, and the intermediate values by affixing to these numbers the fractions ¼, ½, or ¾. so long as these standard specimens are preserved in the institution, so long will instant numerical values for proficiency in writing be maintained. (p. 551).

This Scale Book is an early example of a variable map that plays an essential role in the development of measures that meet the requirements of invariant measurement.

An early example of Thorndike's use of a variable map was in the measurement of the merit of written compositions. In 1916, he wrote a monograph that "consists of one hundred and fifty specimens of English composition whose general merit has been determined with fair precision by a consensus of from 23 to 100 judges" (Thorndike, 1916, p. 1). Within the scaling tradition, objectivity is defined as agreement among judges regarding the ordering by merit of a set of essays during this time period. A good example of this type of scale was developed and published by two of Thorndike's students within the context of writing assessment: Hillegas (1912) and Trabue (1917). Hillegas (1912) proposed a *Scale for the Measurement of Quality in English Composition by Young People*. This scale consists of writing samples whose values had been determined by the median value of a large set of expert judgments. An example of this scale is presented in Figure 5.1. The merit of student writing samples would be matched to these examples located on the scale from low (0: What should I do next Sunday) to high (9: The courage of the panting fugitive ...). This visual display would be recognized today as a variable map (Stone, Wright, & Stenner, 1999). These maps clearly place Thorndike and his students in the scaling tradition.

Thorndike (1904, 1919) described what he considered the five essentials of a valid scale. These five essentials are:

1. objectivity,
2. consistency (unidimensionality),
3. definiteness of facts and their differences from one another,
4. comparability with facts to be measured, and
5. reference to a defined zero point.

He defined objectivity as agreement about the meaning of a scale among competent judges. Consistency was defined in terms of how clearly a set of facts or items could be used to define stable and varying amounts of the same quality (unidimensionality). The third essential of a valid scale proposed by Thorndike addresses the definiteness of the facts or items in terms of how well the location of the items on the scale could be defined with a set of steps or units. Next, Thorndike addressed the importance of being able to use the scale based on the comparability of the facts being measured to the items located on the scale. For example, he was concerned that the user be able to match new writing samples with compositions that had been previously selected to represent locations on an objective scale. Finally, Thorndike argued for the facts to be referenced to a defined zero point, although he recognized that this defined zero point may be absolute or arbitrary. It is clear that these criteria were designed to support and evaluate the types of visual scales and variable maps that he developed with students and colleagues. These essentials of a valid scale were designed to address the special difficulties that Thorndike identified for measurement in the social sciences: "the absence or imperfection of units in which to measure, the lack of constancy in the facts measured, and the extreme complexity of the measurements to be made" (Thorndike, 1919, p. 4).

What I should like to do next Saturday

0.
I went going on to the Dox Saturdays dad day for the boys and I well going home and I well going the boys. I well going a ground road in that my night, and we or night. I well going to shot abouse and I will shoe or the skill of the shen of night.

.001

1.1
I intend to mak a soon man and make an fort and fort smok boll at chidem and hau I whint mn carolyn cob what were mn I will going to the maulns on Saturday.
Georga will come went me.
I whint there whent school on Saturday

1.09

1.9
one next Saturday I expect to go to the city leve next Gaturday to see my cfriend archie king I am going to grow to the baning baiya circus with hims next Saturday fefore I go I have to do my bisd feeding a vrey and hora and chickens and geese next Saturday If I do my work during Easter week vacation I can go to the burning baisy circts with hims

1.83

2.8
Once a pon a time there was a girl. One day she asked me what I was going to do next Saterday so I said, "I am going to go for a swim." And she said, "thats
just where I was going too." next Saterday came we both went down together. We gote home at noon time. after dinner we went to the pictures. There we had a good time. And then came home at night.

2.81

3.8
I would like to go out in the after noon and play catching the ball. Go over to Bertha's house and have a few girls to come with me and be on each others side. I have a tennis ball too play. The game is that one person should stand quite a ways from another person and throw the ball too one then another. Someone then be in the middle and try too get the ball a way from someone then she takes this persons place who she caught the ball from. Then till every person has a chance.

3.81

5.0
Next Saturday I should like to go away and have a good time on a farm. I should like to watch the men plowing the fields and planting corn, wheat, and oats and other things planted on farms. Next Saturday I will go to the Pioneer meeting if nothing happens so that I cannot go. I should like to go swimming but it is not warm enough and I would catch a bad cold. I should like to go to my aunts and drive the horse. I do not drive without some older person with me, so I cannot go very often. I should like to see my aunts cat and her kittens, too. I think I can, to.

4.97

6.0
I should like to join my girl friends, who are going to the city on the 9:25 A. M. train. They are going shopping in the morning and will have lunch to-gether, then they are going to the Hippodrome. After the Hippodrome, they are all going home to dinner to one of the girls houses, she lives on Riverside Drive so they expect to take the "Fifth Avenue Bus" up there. The evening will be devoted to playing games, singing and dancing.

6.01

7.2
If I had a thousand dollars to spend, I think I would take a trip to San Francisco by train with the rest of the family, and keep it as a sea-side hotel. It would be glorious to see the surf again, and to escape from the cold blustering weather of December for the balmy breezes of the ocean, and the whiff of orange blossoms.
We could take long drives under shady trees, visit the orange and olive groves and bathe in the surf. Think of bathing in the ocean in December!
Coming home again I should enjoy stopping at Yellow Stone Park. It would be lots of fun to camp out, and to ride over the prairies on a frisky pony. It would be very interesting to notice the change of climate as we got farther east, and to go to bed on the train one evening feeling warm, and waking up the next morning feeling very chilly.
I am afraid by the time I would get home a thousand dollars would be pretty well used up; but if not I would like to give a party.

7.23

8.0
One Sunday, towards the end of my summer vacation, I was in bathing at the Parkway Baths. In the Brighton Beach Motordrome, a few rods away, an aviation meet was going on. Several times one of its circling machines had gone whirling by over our heads, so that when the buzzing exhaust of a flier was heard it did not cause very much comment. Soon, however, the white planes of "Tom" Sopwith's Wright machine were seen glimmering above the grandstand. Everyone stood spellbound as he circled the track several times and then headed out to sea. He was seen to have a passenger with him. Suddenly, the regular hum of his motor was broken by severe pops, and the engine ran silent. The machine in response to its movements in the big flier tilted and swooped down to the beach from aloft like an eagle. The te ilted crowd made a rush to get out of the way as the airship came on, but Sopwith could not land on the beach, but skimmed along close to the water instead. Suddenly his wing caught the water, and the big machine somersaulted and sank beneath the waves. The aviators soon came bobbing up and were taken away in a launch, but the accident will not soon be forgotten by those who saw it.

8.00

9.0
The courage of the panting fugitive was not gone; she was game to the tip of her high-bred ears, but the fearful pace at which she had just been going told on her. Her legs trembled, and her heart beat like a trip-hammer. She slowed her speed perforce, but still find industriously up the right bank of the stream. When she had gone a couple of miles and the dogs were evidently gaining again, she crossed the broad, deep brook, climbed the steep left bank, and fled on in the direction of the Mt. Marcy trail. The fording of the river threw the hounds off for a time; she knew by their uncertain yelping, as they galloped up and down the opposite bank, that she had a little respite; she could even hear them, as they plashed on until she used, the baying was fainter in her ears, and then she dropped exhausted upon the ground.

Figure 5.1 Hillegas Scale
Hillegas, M.B. A scale for the measurement of quality in English composition by young people. Teachers College, Columbia University, 1912.

2. Absolute Scaling and Psychophysics: Thurstone

... I speculated about the possible use of the new psychophysical toys.
(Thurstone, 1952, p. 310)

Thurstone (1952) was explicit about the connections between psychophysics and psychological measurement. In 1924, he taught a course on psychological measurement at the University of Chicago. It was at this point in time that he introduced the idea that the calibration of stimuli in psychophysics, such as the comparison of weights to a standard weight of 100 grams, could be replaced with more interesting stimuli to compare.

Instead of lifted weights we used a list of offenses presented in pairs with the instruction that they should be judged as to their relative seriousness. The subject checked one of each pair of offenses to indicate which he thought was the more serious. It was now apparent that the classical method of constant stimuli is a special case of the more complete psychophysical method of paired comparison ... by the method of paired comparison we were able to allocate each stimulus to a point on the subjective continuum. (Thurstone, 1952, p. 307)

The method of paired comparisons provided the basis for the calibration of stimulus or items onto a subjective continuum or latent variable. It also formed the basis for Thurstone's law of comparative judgment.

In addition to the use of psychophysics to scale items for attitude measurement, Thurstone also used it to form the basis for scaling test items. The idea and motivation for developing a new method of item scaling occurred to Thurstone while he was "trying to tease out the logic of some well-known educational scales and mental age scales" (1925, p. 433). He found that previous researchers had not provided an adequate description of their methods for the calibration of items. In order to remedy this situation, Thurstone (1925, 1927, 1928) set out his views on items scaling in this series of articles in the 1920s. These articles provide the basis for his method of absolute scaling. According to Thurstone,

It is called an absolute scaling method because it is independent of the scaling unit represented by the raw scores. The unit of measurement is the standard deviation of test ability in any given age group. This distribution is assumed, as usual, to be normal and the base line is an abstract scale of test ability independent of the raw scoring unit. (1928, p. 441)

Engelhard (1984) provides a detailed description of how Thurstone's method of absolute scaling is an approach for achieving person-invariant item calibration.

Thurstone treated issues of item-invariant person measurement from both a group-based approach based on his method of absolute scaling (1925, 1927, 1928a, 1928b), and an individual-based perspective (1926). For the purposes of item-invariant measurement of persons, the method described in Thurstone (1926) has clear connections to current work on person response functions. Engelhard (1991) describes Thurstone's method for item-invariant measurement, and compares his method to approaches suggested by Thorndike and Rasch.

As pointed out by Bock (1997), one of the first glimpses of what would eventually become item response theory can be seen in the work on L.L. Thurstone (1925) in his paper entitled: "A Method of Scaling Psychological and Educational Tests." In this paper, Thurstone calibrated the items from Binet and Simon (1905) onto an age-grade scale and percent of children with correct responses on the y-axis. Empirical item response functions are shown in Figure 5.2. Thurstone used an observed variable on the x-axis (chronological age), and this is eventually replaced in future work with a latent variable on the x-axis designed to represent the construct being measured. Thurstone clearly recognized the close connections between the research in psychophysics by Fechner (1860) and Urban (1908), and successfully took the important steps towards moving measurement away from the test-score traditions into a scaling tradition that can be used to create a visual display of the variable being represented by a set of test items.

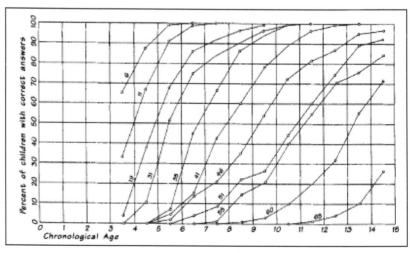

Adapted from Thurstone, L.L. 1925. A method of scaling psychological and educational tests. *Journal of Educational Psychology, 16,* p. 444

Figure 5.2   Proportions of correct response to selected items from the Binet-Simon test among children in successive age groups.

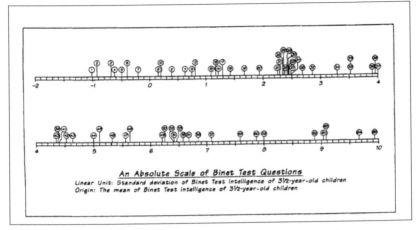

An Absolute Scale of Binet Test Questions
Linear Unit: Standard deviation of Binet Test intelligence of 3½-year-old children
Origin: The mean of Binet Test intelligence of 3½-year-old children

Adapted from Thurstone, L.L. 1925. A method of scaling psychological and educational tests. *Journal of Educational Psychology, 16,* p. 449.

Figure 5.3   Estimated location of items on age scale with arbitrary origin and unit of measurement.

Based on his method of absolute scaling, Thurstone (1925) mapped the Binet items onto a latent variable scale. This is shown in Figure 5.3, and it represents an early variable map with items clearly located on a line based on the data represented in Figure 5.2.

It is also significant that Thurstone's influential little book on attitude measurement had the phrase "psychophysical method" in the subtitle (Thurstone & Chave, 1929). This highlights the connection between psychophysics and modern scaling methods.

It appears that Thurstone never recognized that both items and persons could be simultaneously calibrated onto the same underlying scales. Throughout his publications on absolute scaling, he kept item calibrations separate from the person measurement aspects of his research in psychometrics. It should also be recognized that from the perspective of psychophysics, Thurstone introduced the person into the stimulus-response theme that was dominant in the 1920s (Still, 1987).

Item response theory is described in the next section. One of the major contributions of Georg Rasch was the recognition that item and persons can be mapped onto the same line simultaneously when the requirements of invariant measurement are met.

3. Item Response Theory: Birnbaum and Rasch

The dominant measurement models today are based on item response theory. According to Bock and Moustaki (2007), item response theory (IRT) deals with the statistical analysis of data in which response of each of a number of respondents to each of a number of items or trials are assigned to defined mutually exclusive categories ... IRT was developed mainly in connection with educational measurement, where the main objective is to measure individual student achievement. Prior to the introduction of IRT, the statistical treatment of achievement data was based entirely on what is now referred to as "classical test theory". That theory is predicated on the test score (usually the student's number of correct responses to the items presented) as the observation. (p. 469)

The two IRT models that dominate current practices are based on the work of Birnbaum and Rasch.

Birnbaum

Birnbaum (1968) proposed the use of a cumulative logistic distribution to model the item response function. Earlier researchers working within the IRT tradition included Richardson (1936), Lawley (1943), and Lord (1952). These earlier measurement researchers based their models of the item response function on the normal distribution. This is in contrast to Birnbaum who described a logistic IRT model in a series of publications (Birnbaum, 1957, 1958a, 1958b). His original model included two item characteristics: item difficulty and item discrimination. Later, Birnbaum added a lower asymptote to the item response function in his influential section in Lord and Novick (1968). This lower asymptote has been labeled a "guessing" parameter. One of the distinctive features of the Birnbaum model is that the test scores are replaced by the full response patterns. This has the advantage of capturing all of the information in the full responses provided by persons to a set of items. Among the disadvantages of item-pattern scoring is that the number correct or total score is no longer a sufficient statistic for estimating person location on the latent variable. In other words, each total score can be created by multiple item patterns. For example, a total score of 3 out 4 can be obtained by each of the following patterns: [1 1 1 0], [0 1 1 1], [1 0 1 1], and [1 1 0 1]. This implies that items and persons can no longer be mapped simultaneously onto a single latent variable or construct as represented by a variable map. A major proponent of Birnbaum's model was Fred Lord (1980) who was instrumental in the development of computer programs and the application of Birnbaum's model to solve practical measurement problems.

Rasch

The comparison between two stimuli should be independent of which particular individuals were instrumental for the comparison; and it should also be indepen-

dent of which stimuli within the considered class were or might also have been compared.

Symmetrically, a comparison between two individuals should be independent of which particular stimuli with the class considered were instrumental for the comparison; and it should also be independent of which other individuals were also compared on the same or on some other occasion.

(Rasch, 1961, pp. 331–332)

Rasch also developed an IRT model based on the cumulative logistic distribution (Rasch 1960/1980). He started with a set of requirements that he labeled "specific objectivity" (Rasch, 1977). Rasch's concept of specific objectivity support the view of invariant measurement developed in this book. Rasch's approach allowed the conceptual separation of items and persons, unlike Birnbaum who did not provide a framework for the simultaneous location of both persons and items on the latent variable that can be represented by a variable map. One of the distinctive differences between Rasch and Birnbaum is that Rasch preserved the concept of a summed or total score, while Birnbaum based his work on modeling item response patterns. In other words, raw scores can be obtained by various combinations of item response patterns, and each pattern within the Birnbaum model implies variation in person location on the latent variable or construct. Birnbaum's focus was on the measurement of persons and the development of an ability scale to represent person locations on the latent variable. The use of pattern scoring means that there is one metric and map for the person locations on the scale, while there are multiple item maps for the latent variable that depend on the person's location on the ability scale. For example, with the Birnbaum model, it is necessary in standard setting based on items maps to create a map for each specific response probability because variable maps vary at different points along the scale (Lewis, Mitzel, & Green, 1996). This was illustrated in a previous chapter with crossing item response functions.

Rasch developed his work on measurement theory independently of other research work in psychometrics. Rasch clearly stated his quest for invariant measurement based on his concept of specific objectivity. Invariant measurement was the salient theme in his measurement work. As pointed out numerous times in this book, invariant measurement forms the basis for the new rules of measurement that will dominate measurement in the 21st century. It should be stressed that Rasch described an essential approach that provides the opportunity to meet the requirements for invariant measurement in the human sciences.

A major proponent of Rasch models was Ben Wright, and he was instrumental in the development of computer programs and the application of Rasch models to solve a host of practical measurement problems. According to Wright, "The Rasch model is so simple that its immediate relevance to contemporary measurement practice and its extensive possibilities for solving measurement problems may not be fully apparent" (1977, p. 104).

4. Non-Parametric Item Response Theory: Guttman, Lazarsfeld, and Mokken

Item response theory provides a very general framework for examining responses by persons to a set of items (Bock & Moustaki, 2007). Sijtsma and Meijer (2007) view item response theory as being composed of nonparametric and parametric models. For example, the Birnbaum and Rasch models described in the previous section are considered parametric IRT models from this perspective. Nonparametric item response theory provides an exploratory framework for the analysis of item and person data, while parametric IRT primarily deals with confirmatory data analysis for fitting specific models to data.

Siegel (1956), in his classic work on nonparametric statistics, used the following definition:

[a] nonparametric statistical test is a test whose model does not specify conditions about the parameters of the population from which the sample was drawn. Certain assumptions are associated with most nonparametric statistics tests, i.e., that the observations are independent and that the variable under study has underlying continuity, but these assumptions are fewer and much weaker than those associated with parametric tests. Moreover, nonparametric tests do not require measurement so strong as that required for parametric tests; most nonparametric tests apply to data in an ordinal scale, and some apply also to data in a nominal scale. (p. 31)

Siegel (1956) argued for the appropriate matching of measurement scale (nominal, ordinal, interval, and ratio) with method of statistical analysis. This was the main message that many readers took from his book. However, Siegel was also laying out several larger points related to nonparametric models. He suggested that models can be built without strong assumptions regarding the distributions of population parameters. He also recognized that although weaker assumptions may have less power from a statistical perspective, they can in some cases lead to more general conclusions. According to Sijtsma and Meijer (2007),

the reason for calling one class of IRT models nonparametric and another parametric is that the former only put order restrictions on response functions, and the latter assumes a specific parametric function, such as the logistic or the normal ogive. (p. 720)

Guttman, Lazarsfeld, and Mokken provide nonparametric IRT models without a set of strict requirements regarding the form of the operating characteristic function. Guttman provides a nonparametric IRT model that is deterministic, and that also includes very rigorous requirements. Lazarsfeld and Mokken provide probabilistic versions of nonparametric IRT models. The major distinction between parametric (Rasch and Birnbaum) and non-parametric (Lazarsfeld, Guttman, and Mokken) models is based on whether or not the form of the operating characteristic (OC) function is specified to represent the relationship between the item and person locations with the probability of success on a dichotomous item. Parametric models specify the form of the OC function, such as the logistic function, while non-parametric models estimate the form of the function empirically based on the specific data set being examined.

Guttman

> The Guttman scale is one of the very clearest examples of a good idea in all of psychological measurement. Even with an unsophisticated—but intelligent— consumer of psychometrics, one has only to show him a perfect scale and the recognition is almost instantaneous, "Yes, that's what I want."
>
> (Cliff, 1983, p. 284)

In the 1940s, Louis Guttman (1944, 1950) laid the groundwork for a new technique designed to explore the unidimensionality of a set of test items. According to Guttman (1950),

> One of the fundamental problems facing research workers ... is to determine if the questions asked on a given issue have a single meaning for the respondents. Obviously, if a question means different things to different respondents, then there is no way that the respondents can be ranked ... Questions may appear to express a single thought and yet not provide the same kind of stimulus to different people. (p. 60)

Guttman proposed a set of requirements that can be used to test the hypothesis of unidimensionality. Guttman scaling is the specific technique he recommended for determining whether or not a set of items and group of persons met of the requirements of a Guttman Scale. Guttman scales are also called perfect scales. Guttman determined the requirements of these perfect scales based on an ideal model of a scale. Guttman considered the comparative analysis of the ideal and observed response patterns as a method for identifying individuals or groups for further study. "As a matter of fact, a study of the deviants is an interesting by-product of the scale analysis. Scale analysis actually picks out individuals for case studies" (Guttman, 1944, p. 149). These "deviants" define unexpected cases that may yield important new understandings of both items and persons. The study of deviants and apparently anomalous results can play an important role in scientific progress (Kuhn, 1970).

In essence, Guttman scaling is a technique for examining whether or not a set of items administered to a group of persons is unidimensional. A data matrix (persons by items or persons by categories within items) meets the requirements of Guttman scaling when person scores reproduce the exact item responses in the data matrix. A set of items that meets this condition is defined as a Guttman scale.

Guttman scaling consists of several steps (Engelhard, 2005). First of all, the responses of persons to a set of items are collected. Next, the items are ordered by difficulty and the persons are ordered by the number correct scores. This ordered data matrix defines a Scalogram. The third step is to examine the extent to which ordered data matrix has the distinctive pattern that defines a Guttman scale. For example, a perfect Guttman scale with four items ordered from easy to hard consists of five ideal response patterns reflecting scores of 1 to 4:

0: [0 0 0 0],
1: [1 0 0 0],
2: [1 1 0 0],
3: [1 1 1 0],
4: [1 1 1 1].

All other response patterns, such as [0 1 0 0] are considered inconsistent because a person would get the easy item incorrect, and the second and harder item correct. See Engelhard (2005a) for a detailed description of various methods for examining the model-data fit between perfect Guttman response patterns and observed data matrices.

Guttman scaling is considered a deterministic model, and it provides the prototype for conceptualizing ideal-type models for scales in the social, behavioral, and health sciences. Nunnally (1967) points out that "in spite of the intuitive appeal of the Guttman scale, it is highly impractical" (p. 64). Nunnally (1967) summarized his criticisms of Guttman scales as follows:

> ... the deterministic model underlying the Guttman scale is thoroughly illogical for most psychological measurement because (1) almost no items exist that fit the model, (2) the presence of a triangular pattern is a necessary but not sufficient condition for the fit of the model in particular instances, (3) the triangular pattern can be (and usually is) artificially forced by dealing with a small number of items that vary greatly in difficulty, (4) the model aspires only to develop ordinal scales, and (5) there are better intuitive bases for developing models for psychological attributes. Considering this heavy weight of criticism, it is surprising that some people still consider this deterministic model a good basis for developing measures of psychological attributes. (1967, p. 66)

In response to this criticism, it is important to recognize that Guttman developed his model of scaling as an ideal type to provide a theoretical basis for defining a perfect scale. He was not under the illusion that most items would meet these requirements. He also recognized that the distinctive triangular pattern of a perfect Guttman scale must be used in conjunction with other evidence including item content (universe of attributes). Point 3 is accurate because it is certainly the case that if the item difficulties are more spread out, then the Guttman patterns are more likely to occur. This does not necessarily constitute a flaw in Guttman scaling. In regard to point 4, discussion in the measurement and social science research communities continue regarding the relative value of ordinal scales, and the potential usefulness of nonparametric versus parametric models of measurement data (Cliff & Keats, 2003). Finally, point 5 depends in a fundamental way on philosophical issues regarding measurement in the social sciences, and it is clearly a debatable issue.

Guttman scaling is important because it lays out in a very obvious way many of the issues and requirements that are necessary for the development of a scale. Guttman preferred to limit his approach to scaling to ranks and ordinal-level person measures that reflect a deterministic and non-parametric approach to scaling. Even though his requirements for a perfect scale are imbedded within a deterministic framework, Andrich (1985) has shown how a probabilistic model based on Rasch measurement theory (Rasch, 1960/1980) can achieve many of these theory-based requirements. Andrich (1985) has pointed out the close connections between Guttman's deterministic model and Rasch's probabilistic model.

> ... technical parallels between the SLM [dichotomous Rasch model] and the Guttman scale are not a coincidence. The connections arise from the same essential conditions required in both, including the requirement of invariance of scale and location values with respect to each other. (Andrich, 1988, p. 40)

In addition to the strong relationship between Guttman scaling and Rasch measurement theory, the origins of nonparametric item response theory can be found in Guttman's early work (Mokken, 1971, 1997; Sijtsma & Molenaar, 2002). Mokken scaling has its origins in Guttman scaling.

In practice, sets of items and groups of persons do not meet exactly the requirements of a Guttman scale, but conceptually it provides a useful framework that aids us in thinking about invariant measurement. As pointed out by Stouffer et al. (1950),

> the fact that a perfect Guttman scale is not obtained except approximately is not in itself a denial of the value of the model. The crucial question is whether it has ideal properties from which one may make varied logical deductions ... and whether it leads to rapid and enlightening empirical tests of hypotheses. (p. 7)

When data fit the requirements of Guttman scaling, they have also met the five requirements of invariant measurement. Rasch models can be considered probabilistic versions of Guttman scaling that also meet the five requirements of invariant measurement.

Lazarsfeld

Much of the work on measurement in the human sciences has been contributed by researchers working with disciplinary backgrounds in psychology and education. A notable exception is the sociologist Paul F. Lazarsfeld. During the 1940s and 1950s, Lazarsfeld proposed latent structure analysis as a method for scaling attitude items. Latent structure analysis generalized the Spearman-Thurstone factor analysis models for use with qualitative observations. Guttman during this time period (1940s–1950s) recognized that the methods of factor analysis did not work properly with qualitative observations classified into two categories, and as a response developed Guttman scaling to determine unidimensionality in ordered qualitative data. Lazarsfeld during this same time period took a different approach, and he systematically introduced a new method for factoring qualitative data based on the algebra of dichotomous systems (Lazarsfeld, 1961). A fundamental contribution of Lazarsfeld (1958) was the development and application of the concept of conditional independence.

> the idea of making the principle of local independence the nub of index construction, even of concept formation in the social sciences, is the central logical feature of latent structure analysis. Together with conventional probability notions and some newly developed but quite orthodox algebra, all procedures and all empirical finding derive from it. (Lazarsfeld, 1959, p. 506)

Local independence is one of the critical assumptions of item response theory, and it states that given a person's location on the latent variable, the item responses are statistically independent (Bock & Moustaki, 2007).

Lazarsfeld (1958) stressed that the "process by which concepts are translated into empirical indices has four steps: an initial imagery of the concept, the specification of dimensions, the selection of observable indicators, and the combination of indicators into indices " (p. 109). Lazarsfeld (1958) also recognized the importance of invariant measurement. In his words,

> In the formation of indices of broad social and psychological concepts, we typically select a relatively small number of items from a large number of possible ones suggested by the concept and its attendant imagery. It is one of the notable features of such indices that correlations with outside

variables will usually be about the same, regardless of the specific "sampling" of items which goes into them from the broader group associated with the concept. This rather startling phenomenon has been labeled the "interchangeability of indices." (p. 113)

This quote illustrates his view of item-invariant measurement of persons (interchangeability of indices).

Latent structure analyses consist of several steps. Lazarsfeld (1959) specified nine steps:

Choice and specification of the model, accounting equations specialized for the model, the conditions of reducibility, identifiability, identification, computation: the fitting procedure, evaluation of the fit, the recruitment pattern, and classification with scores. These steps are described in detail in Lazarsfeld (1959), and also in Lazarsfeld and Henry (1968). The major resources for latent structure analyses are Lazarsfeld (1950a, b) and the textbook by Lazarsfeld and Henry (1968). Heinen (1996) includes a modern perspective and appreciation of Lazarsfeld's latent structure and latent class models.

Mokken

> Mokken's nonparametric IRT models ... have been successfully applied to the measurement of a wide variety of latent traits in the domains of psychology, sociology, education, political science, medical research, and marketing.
> (Sijtsma & Molenaar, 2002, p. 6)

Mokken (1971) published an approach to scaling that represents a "generalization of Lazarsfeld's latent structure model (Lazarsfeld, 1959) to multivariate response variables and multidimensional subject and item parameters" (p. 325). In essence, Mokken scaling can be viewed as a nonparametric item response theory model that provides a probabilistic version of Guttman scaling, and that also provides an approach for examining Rasch's requirements for invariant measurement.

> [t]his enabled us to treat in terms of this general model the special requirements imposed by a measurement theory developed by Rasch (1961) which led to models in which *item parameters* were estimated independently of the populations distribution (or selection) of subjects (*population free estimation*), and in which *subjects* are measured (estimated) independently of the particular selection of items (*item selection free*). (Mokken, 1971, p. 325, italics in the original)

One of the essential features of Mokken scaling is that it returned to the lens of duality: item calibration and person measurement viewed as two distinct activities for some purposes. According to Mokken (1971),

... a simple model containing one subject and one item difficulty parameter of a very general form. We introduced the concepts of *monotone homogeneity* for models in which the probability of a positive response *increases* monotonically with the subject parameter. We also introduced the concepts of *double monotony* and *holomorphism* for monotonely homogeneous models in which the probability of a positive response is also monotonically *decreasing* for the item difficulty parameter. (p. 325)

Mokken proposed two models for examining aspects of invariant measurement based on the monotone homogeneity (MH) model that can be used to provide an invariant ordering of persons by total score, and the double monotonicity (DM) model that can also be used to obtain sample-invariant item ordering. Measurement invariance is one of the primary aims of item response theory (Bock & Moustaki, 2007).

A useful resource on Mokken Scaling and non-parametric IRT is Sijstma and Molenaar (2002). Non-parametric models have not been applied as frequently as parametric IRT models to solve practical measurement problems. It is anticipated that the use of nonparametric item response theory will increase in the future.

Discussion and Summary

In sum, I would assert that to move forward efficiently we must first look back – to incorporate and build upon the riches of the past, while avoiding futile paths earlier explored and appropriately abandoned. To dwell on the past is folly: to ignore it is absurdity.

(Jaeger, 1987, p. 13)

This chapter examined two research traditions (test-score and scaling) that offer a useful way of viewing a variety of measurement theories during the 20th century. The test-score tradition, as its name implies, focuses on test scores or summated item responses with the main theme of quantifying measurement error and sources of error variance in measurement. One way to conceive of this theme is to recognize that science can focus on either variant or invariant aspects of measurement. The test-score tradition tends to focus on the variant aspects, while the scaling tradition echoes the theme of this book with the clear goal of seeking invariant measurements in the social, behavioral, and health sciences.

In evaluating this chapter, it is important to keep in mind the following caveats from the historian Larry Cuban:

Historians invent the past. I do not mean that historians invent facts, although they frequently discover new ones; I mean that historians ask questions of the past, analyze the available sources and evidence, and filter the data through their experiences, values and expertise to create their own version of what happened. Because historians are products of their times, and differ one from the other, histories of the same event, era, or institutions will vary. (1990, p. 265)

This chapter and the overall book are designed to stress the importance of invariant measurement, and the dual aspects of this concept regarding item-invariant person measurement and person-invariant item calibration. If invariant measurement is achieved, then it is possible to simultaneously locate both items and persons on variable maps. Variant measurements within the test-score tradition do not yield variable maps.

It is also important to recognize the concept of ideal-type models. Gutt-man, Rasch, and Mokken recognized that the requirements of an ideal measurement model should be specified a priori. These ideal-type models possess a variety of desirable characteristics including invariance. In practice, these ideal-type models become a framework for determining whether or not a particular data set has met these requirements, and also how well they have met these requirements. Ideal-type models provide a strong theoretical basis for measurement in the social, behavioral, and health sciences that allows researchers to construct useful scales and instruments designed to measure the latent variables and constructs of interest.

The distinction between parametric and non-parametric measurement models is another important concept in understanding measurement theories and the quest for invariant measurement. Parametric models specify a priori the form of the operating characteristic functions that connect the item and person characteristics to the probabilities of a set of responses. Nonparametric models on the other hand allow the researcher to select different forms for the operating characteristic functions.

This chapter illustrates the value of doing historical, philosophical, and comparative work on invariant measurement theory. It is primarily a history of how concepts and issues related to two major research traditions played a role in the quest for invariant measurement during the 20th century. These issues are perennial, and most of the major measurement theories addressed these issues in one way or another. Although social, cultural, and political issues play a role in all technological advances (Porter, 1995), the primary thrust of this chapter has been on the history of ideas. The story in this chapter is designed to highlight the ebb and flow of conceptual frameworks as defined through the lens of research traditions and selected measurement theories. The ideas in this chapter and throughout the book dominated measurement in the human sciences in the 20th century, and they will continue to be sources of discussion and debate in the 21st century. This chapter provides a brief introduction to the history of measurement theory and highlights some of the key ideas of selected measurement theorists.

It is important to develop a clear perspective on how assessment has been viewed during the past 100 years or so. A detailed historical analysis can provide an emergent framework for understanding how much progress or lack of progress has been made in the conceptual and theoretical ideas regarding the practice of assessment. This historical view can help to frame current issues on assessment, and also to suggest areas for future research and policy improvements in educational practices related to assessment an important component of educational policy in contemporary societies. It should be recognized that this historical analysis represents a preliminary exploration of these issues and is limited by this broad scope.

Chapter 6

The Quest for Invariant Measurement within the Scaling Tradition

A major weakness common to both classical test theory and generalizability theory is the sample-dependent nature of the estimation procedures ... one of the critical properties of the item response theories ... is that item parameters are invariant across groups of examinees while at the same time estimates of examine ability or trait level are invariant across sets of items measuring the same ability or trait.

(Messick, 1983, p. 513)

The purpose of this chapter is to continue the historical, philosophical, and comparative discussion on invariant measurement started in the previous chapter. As pointed out by Messick (1983) in the above quote, item response theories within the scaling tradition have the potential to form the basis for invariant measurement. The focus of this chapter is primarily on the scaling tradition that includes item response theories and is a continuation of the historical issues considered in Chapter 5. The previous chapter focused on a general view of measurement theories and presented a general framework for considering measurement theories during the 20th century in terms of two broad research traditions: test-score and scaling traditions.

This chapter provides a detailed look at selected measurement theories within the scaling tradition. The emphasis is on providing a comparative framework to conceptualize how various measurement theorists sought to address issues related to invariant measurement. The quest for invariant measurement of persons and calibration of items is a major underlying goal of the theorists described and analyzed in this chapter. There is a long tradition in the sciences of seeking invariance, and, as Isaacson (2007) stressed in his biography of Albert Einstein, "beneath all of his theories, including relativity, was a quest for invariants ... and the goal of science was to discover it" (p. 3).

It is useful to consider invariant measurement in terms of three general aspects: items, persons and variable maps. Item-invariant measurement of persons includes a consideration of person response functions with a determination of whether or not differential person functioning is occurring based on an examination of person fit. The second aspect concerns the person-invariant calibration of items which includes estimation of item response functions with analyses of differential item functioning or measurement invariance as it is sometimes called (Milsap, 2007). The final aspect is the creation and use of variable maps (Stone, Wright, & Stenner, 1999). If item-invariant person measurement and person-invariant item calibration are accomplished to a satisfactory degree, then it is possible to create a visual display with the locations of both items and persons on an underlying latent variable. This is very desirable—a variable map represents both persons and items located on a construct of interest, and variable maps represent the sin qua non of invariant measurement.

This chapter describes issues related to the three aspects of invariant measurement in detail. The measurement theories of Thorndike, Thurstone, Birnbaum, Rasch, Guttman, Lazarsfeld, and Mokken are analyzed. As pointed out by S.S. Stevens, "...the scientist is usually looking for invariance whether he knows it or not" (1951, p. 20), and these particular measurement theorists placed a very strong emphasis on aspects of both item-invariant person measurement and person-invariant item calibration.

In the first section, the general issues guiding the comparisons among the scaling theories are considered. Next, the focus turns to a description and comparison of measurement theories within the scaling tradition that played an important role in the quest for invariant measurement. A set of important measurement issues are presented, and they are used to frame the comparisons between measurement theories discussed in this chapter. These sections are organized around the categorization of the measurement models as parametric (Thorndike, Thurstone, Birnbaum, and Rasch), and nonparametric (Guttman, Lazarsfeld, and Mokken) with issues related to item-invariant person measurement and person-invariant item calibration addressed for both parametric and nonparametric models. Next, the concept of operating characteristic functions is revisited for each model. The penultimate section in this chapter discusses variable maps. In the final section, a summary and discussion of the main points of the chapter are presented.

General Issues Guiding the Comparisons among the Scaling Theories

It is argued in this chapter and the previous one that a systematic study of the underlying history and philosophy of science is necessary for understanding progress in measurement in the social, behavioral and health sciences. The concept of research traditions (Laudan, 1977) that is similar to paradigms (Kuhn, 1970) is used to guide the description and comparison of various measurement theories. Chapter 5 described two research traditions in measurement theory: test-score and scaling traditions. The test-score tradition does not provide a system for obtaining invariant measurement. In fact, the focus is on variant aspects of the measurement process, such as the estimation of error variances and various reliability coefficients that are sample dependent. The scaling tradition on the other hand does provide the opportunity to meet the requirements of invariant measurement. Measurement theories in the scaling tradition include various item response theories that focus on the invariant aspects of measurement situations.

Within the scaling tradition, there are two major types of models that can be broadly classified as parametric and nonparametric (Sijtsma & Molenaar, 2002). Put simply, parametric models define an underlying parametric structure for the operating characteristic function that relates the probability of an item response to item and person locations on a latent variable. Nonparametric models on the other hand do not specify the parametric form of the operating characteristic function. As pointed in an earlier chapter, the operating characteristic functions can be specified separately for person response and item response functions. Another important idea within the scaling tradition is the duality of person measurement and item calibration (Mosier, 1940, 1941). In essence, the idea of duality reflects whether or not the measurement theorist developed a model that simultaneously parameterized the relationships between person and item locations or treated person measurement and item calibration as separate and conceptually distinct activities.

This section organizes the measurement theories of the scaling tradition based on whether they represent parametric or nonparametric scaling models. It also compares and contrasts how these measurement theorists proposed modeling item-invariant person measurement and person-invariant item calibration. As pointed out earlier, variable maps require both forms of invariance. For the purposes of this chapter, the measurement theorists are classified as follows:

Scaling Tradition

Parametric Models	Nonparametric Models
Thorndike	Guttman
Thurstone	Lazarsfeld
Birnbaum	Mokken
Rasch	

Item-Invariant Person Measurement

It has been well known since the turn of the 20th century that item difficulty influences the meaning and inferences that can be drawn from test scores. Thorndike (1904) recognized that person scores on a test composed of easy items is not equivalent to scores on a test composed of difficult items. According to Thorndike (1904),

If one attempts to measure even so simple a thing as spelling, one is hampered by the fact that there exist no units in which to measure. One may arbitrarily make up a list of words and observe ability by the number spelled correctly. But if one examines such a list one is struck by the inequality of the units. All results based on the equality of any one word with any other are necessarily inaccurate. (p. 7)

The idea that the measurement of persons should be independent of the particular items used to assign a test score has emerged repeatedly. Item-invariant measurement of persons has been sought by several measurement theorists. In order to explore this issue of item-invariant measurement of persons, this section focuses on four measurement theorists (Thorndike, Thurstone, Birnbaum, and Rasch) and the approaches that they used to locate persons on a line that would be independent of the particular items used. In approaching this problem, it is helpful to use the concept of person response functions. From this perspective, a more able person must always have a better chance of success on an item than a less able person: non-crossing person response functions. When invariance is not achieved, then it is useful to examine lack of invariance through the lens of differential person response functions and various forms of person fit indices. Issues related to model-data fit are addressed in Chapter 8.

I. Parametric Models: Thorndike, Thurstone, Birnbaum, and Rasch

Table 6.1 summarizes the perspectives of Thorndike, Thurstone, Birnbaum, and Rasch in terms of fourteen issues related to item-invariant measurement of persons. The measurement models of these four theorists are classified as parametric.

There is general consensus among these theorists on the first six issues. These points of agreement include the recognition of item-invariant measurement as a significant problem in measurement and scaling theory. Each theorist considered the requirements that must be met by a measurement theory in order to achieve item-invariant person measurement. In addressing the Issues 1 and 2, these theorists utilized the concept of a latent variable to represent the construct being measured (Issue 3), and this frequently included the use of person response functions. A comparative perspective on PRFs for these measurement theorists is presented in later section in this chapter.

The underlying structure of the models (Issue 3) exhibits a minor difference with the use of the normal ogive by Thorndike and Thurstone, while Birnbaum and Rasch used the logistic ogive. As pointed out by Birnbaum (1968), the substitution of the logistic ogive for the normal ogive has mathematical advantages, and the two distributions differ by less than .01 (Haley, 1952). There was also general consensus among these four theorists regarding

Table 6.1   Comparison of Measurement Theorists on Major Issues Related to Item-Invariant Measurement of Persons: Parametric Scaling Models

Issues	Thorndike	Thurstone	Birnbaum	Rasch
1 Recognized importance of item-invariant measurement of individuals	Yes	Yes	Yes	Yes
2 Identified requirements of item-invariant measurement	Yes	Yes	Yes	Yes
3 Structure of model	Probabilistic, parametric (normal)	Probabilistic, parametric (normal	Probabilistic, parametric (logistic)	Probabilistic, parametric (logistic)
4 Utilized latent variable concept	Yes	Yes	Yes	Yes
5 Avoided use of total-score metric	Yes	Yes	Yes (Pattern scores)	Yes
6 Used person response functions	Yes	Yes	Yes	Yes
7 Ideal-type model	No	No	No	Yes
8 Model-data fit	Model to *data*	Model to *data*	Model to *data*	Data to *model*
9 Examined deviations from model	Flagged inconsistent responses	Flagged inconsistent responses	Approach not specified or view unknown	Flagged inconsistent responses
10 Item calibration	Separate process	Separate process	Separate process	Simultaneous process
11 Variable map	Yes	Yes	No	Yes
12 Level of measurement	Interval	Interval	Ordinal	Interval
13 Level of analysis	Group level	Group level	Individual level	Individual level
14 Assumed distribution	Normal	Normal	None required	None required

the avoidance of the use of total scores or summed scores based on number of correct items. This reflected the recognition that items did not provide equal or useful units because they vary in difficulty. Birnbaum's approach was a bit different in the sense that he modeled the full response patterns for persons rather than transforming total scores into useful metrics based on person scores.

There is less agreement among Thorndike, Thurstone, Birnbaum, and Rasch on the next set of six issues (Issues 7–12). Issues 7, 8, and 9 are related to whether or not the theorist viewed measurement from the perspective of an ideal-type model. Ideal-type models specify in detail the requirements that must be met by observed data in order to realized invariant measurement. Rasch was the only theorist in this group that viewed his models explicitly in terms of the requirements necessary for achieving his version of invariant measurement that he called specific objectivity. As pointed out by Andrich (1989),

> The view that the model should be fitted to the data, rather than the other way around, where the model is not chosen capriciously, has profound consequences for the psychometric research agenda. In the traditional approach, the agenda is to search for models that best account for the data. That tends to be carried out by statisticians ... [Rasch measurement] leads to a search for qualitative understandings of why some responses do not accord with the model. That task needs to be carried out by researchers who understand the substance of the variables. (p. 15)

This implies a philosophical position (Issue 8) regarding whether or not models are fit to *data* (statistical perspective) or data are fit to *models* (measurement perspective underlying invariant measurement). This also relates to the approach taken for examining residuals and flagging observations that are not in accordance with the measurement model (Issue 9).

Issue 10 (Item calibration) and Issue 11 (Variable map) are related. Thorndike, Thurstone, and Birnbaum tended to view item calibration and person measurement as separate processes, while Rasch created a measurement model that provides for simultaneous calibration of items and measurement of persons. When calibration and measurement are viewed as separate processes, it is not always possible to simultaneously map both items and persons on to the variable map without additional assumptions. It is possible to create item maps separately for Thorndike, Thurstone, and Rasch, but Birnbaum item maps require the additional specification of a particular response probability as found in the literature on standard setting related to the Bookmark method (Mitzel, Lewis, Patz, & Green, 2001). One of the consequences of this aspect of Birnbaum's model is that the level of measurement (Issue 12) can be considered ordinal, while the other theorists in this section provide person measures with interval-level characteristics. Thorndike and Thurstone focused primarily on groups as the level of analysis (Issue 13), while Birnbaum and

Rasch deliberately created measurement models to represent the responses of individual persons to a set of test items. The distinction between using groups versus individuals as the level of analysis has implications for the assumed distribution of persons on the latent variable. Thorndike and Thurstone tended to use the normal distribution as the reference distribution, while both Birnbaum and Rasch did not have specific requirements for a reference distribution (Issue 14).

2. Non-Parametric Models: Guttman, Lazarsfeld, and Mokken

Table 6.2 summarizes the perspectives of Guttman, Lazarsfeld, and Mokken in terms of the same fourteen issues presented in Table 6.1 related to item-invariant measurement of persons. The measurement models of these three theorists are classified as non-parametric.

Guttman, Lazarsfeld, and Mokken were in general agreement on Issues 1 and 2. Lazarsfeld (1966) did not stress invariance as strongly as the others in this section, but he clearly recognized and valued invariance over subsets of items. In his words,

In the formation of indices of broad social and psychological concepts, we typically select a relatively small number of items … it is one of the notable features of such indices that correlation with outside variables usually will be about the same, regardless of the specific "sampling" of items that goes into them from the broader group associated with the concept. This rather startling phenomenon has been labeled "the interchangeability of indices." (p. 190)

All three of the scaling models in this section are considered nonparametric (Issue 3) with Guttman's model defined in a deterministic fashion rather than a stochastic or probabilistic form that undergirds Lazarsfeld's approach to Latent Structure Analysis (LSA; 1950a), and also Mokken scaling. Mokken scaling provides a link between LSA and Rasch measurement models (Mokken, 1971).

Issue 4 is also related to the structure of the model. It appears that Guttman used the idea of a latent variable in an implicit fashion, while the use of trace lines (another name for item response functions) and latent traits was explicit in the measurement theories of Lazarsfeld and Mokken. Lazarsfeld avoided the use of the total-score metric (Issue 5), while Guttman and Mokken advocated for the development of meaningful metrics for the total-score scale. For example, Guttman patterns provide one way to make the total-score scale meaningful by defining the specific items answered correctly or endorsed by persons with each total score. On Issue 6, Guttman and Lazarsfeld did not explicitly use person response functions, and it is not clear whether or not Mokken used this concept. As pointed out in the previous section, ideal-type models (Issue

Table 6.2   Comparison of Measurement Theorists on Major Issues Related to
Item-Invariant Measurement of Persons: Non-Parametric Scaling Models

	Issues	*Guttman*	*Lazarsfeld*	*Mokken*
1	Recognized importance of item-invariant measurement of persons	Yes	Yes (scale exchangeability)	Yes
2	Identified requirements of item-invariant measurement	Yes	Yes	Yes
3	Structure of model	Deterministic (nonparametric)	Probabilistic (nonparametric)	Probabilistic (nonparametric)
4	Utilized latent variable concept	Yes (Implicit)	Yes (Trace lines)	Yes
5	Avoided use of total-score metric	No	Yes	No
6	Used person response functions	No	No	Approach not specified or view unknown
7	Ideal-type model	Yes	No	Yes
8	Model-data fit	Data to *model*	Model to *data*	Data to *model*
9	Examined deviations from model	Major focus of model	Approach not specified or view unknown	Designed to take focus off Guttman errors
10	Item calibration	Simultaneous process	Separate process	Simultaneous with separate issues
11	Variable map	Yes (scalogram)	No	Yes
12	Level of measurement	Ordinal	Ordinal	Ordinal
13	Level of analysis	Individual level	Group level	Individual level
14	Assumed distribution	None required	None required	None required

7) specify the requirements of invariant measurement a priori. Guttman clearly viewed his approach to measurement in terms of an ideal-type model, while Lazarsfeld developed data-based models. Mokken scaling bridged the gap between a pure ideal-type model, and measurement models with relaxed requirements that allowed examining separately whether or not item-invariant measurement and person-invariant calibration have been accomplished. It is clear that both Guttman and Mokken tended to stress the model over the data, while Lazarsfeld reflected more of a statistical perspective of fitting models to

data with data being privileged over the measurement model. Issue 9 is also related to Issues 7 and 8—a concern with ideal-type models and fitting data to a particular measurement model leads directly to a concern with residual analyses that examine the fit between the data and the model. Guttman scaling places examination of these deviations in a central role, and in fact Mokken scaling, as well as Rasch scaling, take the focus of the measurement model off Guttman errors (Engelhard, 2005a).

Guttman and Mokken viewed item calibration (Issue 10) as a simultaneous process in conjunction with person measurement with the added distinction that Mokken allowed the option for addressing the calibration and measurement separately at early stages of the development of a measurement scale. Lazarsfeld viewed item calibration and person measurement as separate processes. When item calibration and person measurement are viewed as a simultaneous process, then it is possible to create variable maps with the locations of both item and persons on the same scale. Both Guttman and Mokken scales can yield variable maps (Issue 11), while Lazarsfeld's latent structure analysis does not offer this type of visual display and understanding of the latent variable. It is interesting to consider that Guttman's Scalogram analysis provides another type of visual display that can be considered a type of variable map.

In terms of Issue 12 (Level of measurement), all three measurement theorists in this section created scaling models that yield ordinal-level measurement. Lazarsfeld focused on groups as the level of analysis (Issue 13), while both Guttman and Mokken developed scaling models with the individual as the level of analysis. None of the models in this section require an assumed distribution of item locations (Issue 14).

Person-Invariant Item Calibration

Person-invariant item calibration and scaling of test scores has been a long standing problem for measurement in social, behavioral and health sciences. The idea that measures should be independent of the particular persons used to develop the scales has emerged repeatedly. Person-invariant calibration of items has been sought by several measurement theorists. In order to explore this issue, this section continues the discussion with four measurement theorists presented in the previous section (Thorndike, Thurstone, Birnbaum, and Rasch) and examines the approaches that they used to locate items on a line that would be independent of the particular persons used. Item response functions provide a way to frame the issue of person-invariant item calibration. From this perspective, a person must always have a better chance of success on an easy item than a hard item: non-crossing item response functions. When invariance is not achieved, then it is useful to examine lack of invariance through the lens of differential item response functions and various forms of item fit indices that are described in Chapter 8. Milsap (2007) defines measurement invariance as follows:

At its root, the notion of measurement invariance (MI) is that some properties of a measure should be independent of the characteristics of the person being measured, apart from those characteristics that are the intended focus of the measure. (p. 462)

I. Parametric Models: Thorndike, Thurstone, Birnbaum, and Rasch

Table 6.3 summarizes the issues related to the sample-invariant calibration of items for measurement theorists using parametric IRT models. Since there is a duality between person measurement and item calibration, these issues are comparable to those shown in Table 6.1 with the focus of this section on person-invariant calibration of items.

Thorndike, Thurstone, Birnbaum, and Rasch had comparable concerns with the first six issues in Table 6.3. Issue 5 reflects whether or not the measurement theorists used a non-linear transformation of the percent-correct metric to calibrate items. Thorndike, Thurstone, and Rasch used a set of related transformations of the percent-correct metric called probable errors (normit transformation divided by .6745), normal deviates (normit transformation), logits (logistic transformation), while Birnbaum built his scoring model around pattern scores.

There is also good agreement on the next six issues (Issues 7–12) with three exceptions. First of all, Rasch viewed item calibration and person measurement as simultaneous processes, while the other measurement theorists in this section viewed the item calibration as separate from person measurement. The second difference is on Issue 11 (variable map). As pointed out earlier, Birnbaum's scaling model does not produce an invariant ordering of items on the latent variable. The order of the item difficulties vary as a function of person location on the latent variable. The final difference is that Birnbaum scaling produces ordinal level measurement, while Thorndike, Thurstone, and Rasch measurement models offer the opportunity to achieve interval level scales (Issue 12).

The last two issues in Table 6.3 are related with Thorndike and Thurstone using a group level of analysis (Issue 13) with the assumption of a normal distribution (Issue 14), while Birnbaum and Rasch measurement models focus on the individual as the level of analysis with no distributional assumptions.

2. Non-parametric Models: Guttman, Lazarsfeld, and Mokken

Table 6.4 summarizes the issues related to the sample-invariant calibration of items for measurement theorists using non-parametric IRT models. As was pointed in the previous sections, these issues are similar to those listed in Table 6.2 with the focus switched to item calibration in this section.

Guttman and Mokken both recognized the importance of person-invariant calibration of items (Issue 1), and they discussed requirements for achieving

Table 6.3   Comparison of Measurement Theorists on Major Issues Related to Person-Invariant Calibration of Items: Parametric Scaling Models

	Issues	Thorndike	Thurstone	Birnbaum	Rasch
1	Recognized importance of person-invariant calibration of items	Yes	Yes	Yes	Yes
2	Identified requirements of person-invariant item calibrations	Yes	Yes	Yes	Yes
3	Structure of model	Probabilistic (parametric: normal curve)	Probabilistic (parametric: normal curve)	Probabilistic (parametric: logistic curve)	Probabilistic (parametric: logistic curve)
4	Utilized latent variable concept	Yes	Yes	Yes	Yes
5	Avoided use of total-score metric	Probable errors (PE units)	Normal deviates (SD units)	Pattern scores	Logits (SD units)
6	Used item response functions	Yes	Yes	Yes	Yes
7	Ideal-type model	No	No	No	Yes
8	Model-data fit	Model to *data*	Model to data	Model to *data*	Data to *model*
9	Examined deviations from model	Yes	*Yes*	Yes	Yes
10	Person measurement	Separate process	Separate process	Separate process	Simultaneous process
11	Variable Map	Yes	Yes	No	Yes
12	Level of measurement	Interval	Interval	Ordinal	Interval
13	Level of analysis	Group level	Group level	Individual level	Individual level
14	Assumed distribution	Normal	Normal	None required	None required

Table 6.4   Comparison of Measurement Theorists on Major Issues Related to Person-Invariant Calibration of Items: Non-Parametric Scaling Models

	Issues	*Guttman*	*Lazarsfeld*	*Mokken*
1	Recognized importance of person-invariant calibration of items	Yes	Approach not specified or view unknown	Yes
2	Identified requirements of person-invariant item calibrations	Yes	Approach not specified or view unknown	Yes
3	Structure of model	Deterministic (nonparametric)	Probabilistic (nonparametric)	Probabilistic (nonparametric)
4	Utilized latent variable concept	Yes (Implicit)	Yes	Yes
5	Avoided use of total-score metric	No	Yes	No
6	Used item response functions	Yes (Implicit)	Yes	Yes
7	Ideal-type model	Yes	No	Yes
8	Model-data fit	Data to *model*	Model to *data*	Data to *model*
9	Examined deviations from model	Major focus of model	Approach not specified or view unknown	Designed to take focus off Guttman errors
10	Person measurement	Simultaneous process	Separate process	Simultaneous process, but separable
11	Variable map	Yes	Approach not specified or view unknown	Yes
12	Level of measurement	Ordinal	Ordinal	Ordinal
13	Level of analysis	Individual level	Group level	Individual level
14	Assumed distribution of ability	None required	None required	None required

this goal (Issue 2) in their research. It is more difficult to determine Lazarsfeld's perspectives on these two issues. Lazarsfeld did appreciate Rasch's contributions to invariant measurement: "Rasch has noted that he chose this function [Rasch model] simply because it was very convenient for his purposes; it turned out to be a very sound choice indeed" (Lazarsfeld & Henry, 1968, p. 223). Additional research is needed to clarify Lazarsfeld's views. All three of these theorists used nonparametric models with Guttman using a deterministic framework, while Guttman and Mokken used a probabilistic framework.

As pointed out in the previous section on these theorists, Lazarsfeld and Mokken used the concept of a latent variable with Guttman scaling utilizing this concept implicitly (Issue 4). Lazarsfeld did not use the total-score metric (Issue 5), while both Guttman and Mokken developing scaling models that created useful frameworks for developing meaningful total-score metrics. Item response functions (Issue 6) undergird the measurement models of all three theorists.

Guttman scaling can be viewed as an ideal-type model (Issue 7), and so can Mokken scaling. Ideal-type models imply fitting data to *models* (Issue 8), and then conducting a detailed and systematic examination of deviations from the measurement model (Issue 9). Lazarsfeld models were not ideal-type models (Issue 7), since he emphasized fitting models to *data*. It is not clear how Lazarsfeld approached issues related to the analysis of deviations from the models. Mokken scaling was deliberately designed to take the focus off the deterministic deviations based on the Guttman scaling in order to add a probabilistic model that provided another way to conceptualize lack of model-data fit.

Guttman and Mokken viewed item calibration and person measurement as simultaneous processes (Issue 10) with Mokken suggesting that for some purposes the processes can be treated separately. Lazarsfeld viewed the processes separately. Variable maps (Issue 11) can be created with both Guttman and Mokken scaling, but it is not clear how Lazarsfeld conceptualized Issue 11.

Guttman, Lazarsfeld, and Mokken models yield ordinal level measures (Issue 12). Lazarsfeld models focused on the group as the level of analysis (Issue 13), while Guttman and Mokken used the individual or person as the level of analysis. Since these three models are nonparametric, the form of the distributions of ability (Issue 14) does not need to be specified.

Operating Characteristic Functions

This section focuses in detail on the operating characteristic functions that undergird the measurement models presented in this chapter. The reader should recall that "the operating characteristic of the item response on the discrete response level is the conditional probability function of the item response, given the latent [variable]" (Samejima, 1983, p. 160). For example, Rasch (1960/1980) proposed using the cumulative distribution function of the logistic distribution as the operating characteristic function for modeling dichotomous data. Item response functions represent the probability of a positive set of responses as a function of person locations on the latent variable, while person response functions reflect the probability of a positive set of responses as a function of item locations on the latent variable. The next two sections focus on presenting illustrations of item response functions and person response functions for the seven measurement theorists described in this chapter.

I. Item Response Functions

Item response functions represent the relationship between response probabilities for an item and a group of persons. The concept of an item response function has a long history for measurement theorists working in the scaling tradition. Figure 6.1 provides illustrations to represent Thurstone, Birnbaum, and Rasch, while Figure 6.2. presents the item response functions for the nonparametric models: Guttman, Lazarsfeld, and Mokken. No visual display for item response functions has been found at this time to illustrate Thorndike's model.

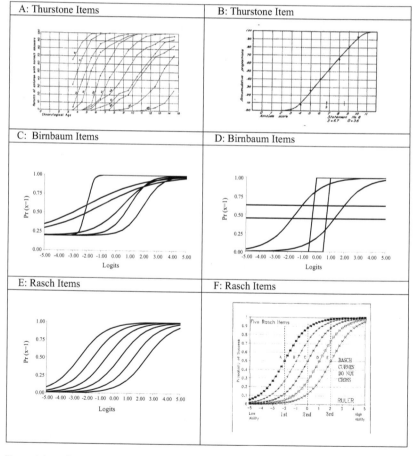

Figure 6.1   Illustrative item response functions (Parametric).

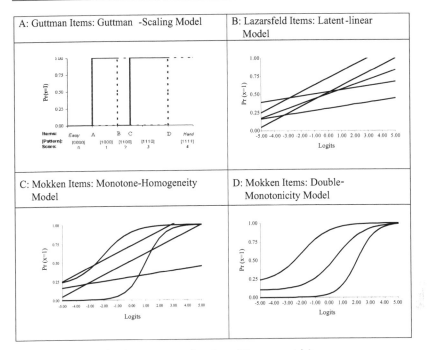

A: Guttman Items: Guttman -Scaling Model	B: Lazarsfeld Items: Latent-linear Model
C: Mokken Items: Monotone-Homogeneity Model	D: Mokken Items: Double-Monotonicity Model

Figure 6.2   Illustrative item response functions (Nonparametric).

One of the earliest visual representations of an item response function is given by Thurstone (1925) and is based on proportions of correct responses to selected items from the Binet-Simon test among children in successive age groups. This display is shown in Panel A of Figure 6.1. At this point in the history of measurement, Thurstone (1925) used an observed variable (age groups) that would later be replaced by a latent variable or construct. Panel B presents an item response function that uses a latent variable (attitude scale) as the x-axis and the accumulative proportion is plotted on the y-axis based on Thurstone and Chave (1929). It should also be noted that at this point in time Thurstone was using the normal ogive to model item response functions.

In Figure 6.1, Panels C and D provide examples of Birnbaum items. It should be recalled that Birnbaum replaced the normal ogive function with the logistic function. As can be seen in these two panels, the forms of these two functions are virtually identical. It should also be noted that Birnbaum items intersect. This crossing of item response functions implies that persons can be ordered, while item order varies as a function of person location on the latent variable scale. The implication of this for variable maps is that invariant item maps cannot be constructed. This is illustrated later in this chapter. Panels E and F show the item response functions for the dichotomous Rasch model. Rasch items do not have intersecting item response functions.

Figure 6.2 gives the item response functions for Guttman, Lazarsfeld, and Mokken items. Guttman items are shown in Panel A. Guttman items have a distinctive step shape based on the deterministic form of the Guttman-scaling model. Lazarsfeld items are shown in Panel B for his latent-linear model. Lazarsfeld used other forms for the item response functions, and this is just one version of his model. Panels C and D illustrate Mokken items based on the Monotone-Homogeneity Model (Panel C), and the Double-Monotonicity Model (Panel D). These two panels clearly illustrate how Mokken items cross under the Monotone-Homogeneity Model, while the Double-Monotonicity Model meets the requirements of monotonically increasing and non-intersecting item response functions. When the item response functions cross, then it is not possible to simultaneously display both item and person locations on variable maps.

2. Person Response Functions

Person response functions represent the relationship between response probabilities for a set of items by a single person. Figure 6.3 presents a set of person response functions based on the measurement models of Thorndike (1904), Thurstone (1926), Birnbaum (Trabin & Weiss, 1979), and Rasch (1960/1980). Panel A shows a representation of within person variability presented by Thorndike (1904). In response to a set of addition problems, Person S had

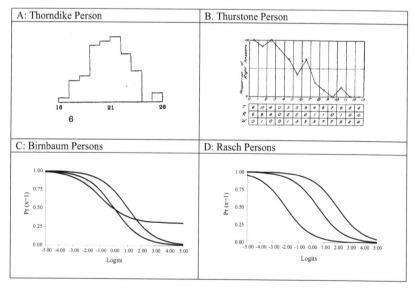

Figure 6.3   Illustrative person response functions (Parametric).

the following distribution of time (in seconds) to solve a series of addition problems:

TABLE XI.

ABILITY IN ADDITION S.

Quantity. Seconds	Frequency.
16–16.9	1
17	5
18	6
19	13
20	14
21	15
22	11
23	7
24	0
25–25.9	2
Total number of measures taken.	74

(Thorndike, 1904, p. 26)

Panel A gives the frequency function for Person S that can also be viewed as the density function for the measurement of individual differences. This density function can be used to represent a person response function for this person. The figure below presents both the frequency function (Person Response Function) and the distribution

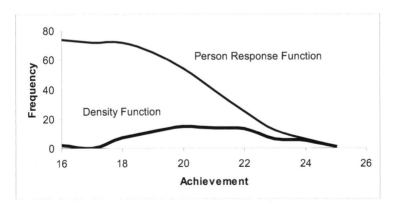

function (Density Function) for the Thorndike (1904) arithmetic data for Person S. The person response function shows how the frequency decreases as difficulty of addition tasks increases. These functions can also be presented as probability distribution and probability density functions by calculating the probabilities that correspond to each frequency.

Thurstone conceptualized person response functions as an approach for scoring individual performance (Panel B). Engelhard (1991) describes Thurstone's approach in detail. Panel C displays the underlying person response function for the Birnbaum model. Finally, Panel D in Figure 6.3 gives rendition of person response functions based on the Rasch model.

Figure 6.4 illustrates the underlying person response functions for the measurement models of Guttman, Lazarsfeld, and Mokken. Panel A illustrates the person response functions for three Guttman persons, while Panel B presents the person response functions for three Lazarsfeld persons based on his latent linear curves (Lazarsfeld, 1960).

Mokken scales are a "generalization of Lazarsfeld's latent structure model" (Mokken, 1971, p. 325), and they provide a framework for merging Lazarsfeld and Rasch models by relaxing some of the requirements of invariant measurement. Mokken (1971) proposed two scaling models: (a) a Monotone-Homogeneity (MH) Model in which the probability of a positive item responses increase monotonically with the person parameters, and (b) a Double-Monotonicity (DM) model in which the probability of a positive

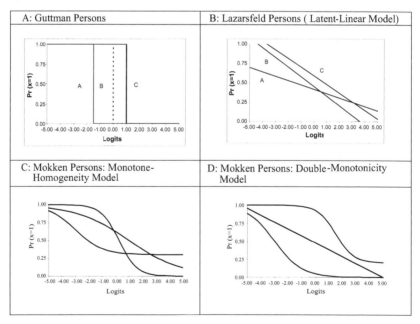

Figure 6.4   Illustrative person response functions (Nonparametric).

response is monotonically increasing, and also the item response functions do not intersect (Sijtsma & Molenaar, 2002). Panel C illustrates three person response functions where the Monotone-Homogeneity (MH) Model holds, and the items can be used to order persons by total score. Both the Rasch and Birnbaum models meet the requirements of the MH Model. Panel D illustrates three person response functions where the DM Model holds, and items and persons can both be ordered on the latent variable. The DM models meet the requirements of invariant measurement.

Variable Maps

An important aspect of invariant measurement involves the location of both items and persons simultaneously on a single underlying latent variable that is called a *variable map*. A variable map provides an organizing concept for viewing the outcomes of a measurement process. Variable maps provide visual displays of the underlying latent variable. It is safe to say that one of the major goals of invariant measurement is to create variable maps with both items and persons located simultaneously on this map. Yardsticks and thermometers are familiar examples of what most people think of as measuring instruments. It is also possible in the social, behavioral, and health sciences to develop "yardsticks" that can be used to represent the important latent variables and constructs that researchers use to represent key ideas regarding how the world works.

Variable maps can be composed of either item maps, person maps or both maps combined and presented simultaneously. The measurement theorists discussed in this chapter had varied views on variable maps. The ideal variable map from the point of view of invariant measurement is to locate both item and persons on the line simultaneously. Item and person maps can be created separately as they were in the early history of the scaling tradition by Thorndike and Thurstone. Rasch calibrated items and measured persons at the same time, and he provided the clearest perspective on invariant measurement. As pointed out earlier in this chapter, Birnbaum's model provides person maps. It is not possible with the Birnbaum model to develop item maps without the specification of additional information, such as the response probability. Guttman scaling can be used to create deterministic variable maps. Mokken scaling offers an intermediate step for achieving invariant measurement that relaxes some of the requirements of invariant measurement. Mokken suggests that measures can later be refined to meet the stricter requirements of Rasch measurement.

Figure 6.5 provides examples of Thorndike variable maps for three content areas: English composition (Hillegas, 1912), Arithmetic (Woody, 1920), and Language (Trabue, 1916). Each panel in Figure 6.5 shows the underlying line or variable map with the items calibrated onto the map. Figure 6.6 gives

A. English composition

Fig. 1. Graphic representation of the relative values of the samples composing the scale. The numbers above the line represent the various unit points in the scale. The numbers below the line represent sample compositions and show their relative positions on the scale. Thus, sample 580 is at the zero point, sample 595 is between the values of 100 and 200, etc.

Sample 580. **Value o.** Artificial sample.

Letter.

Dear Sir: I write to say that it aint a square deal Schools is I say they is I went to a school. red and gree green and brown aint it hito bit I say he don't know his business not today nor yeaterday and you know it and I want Jennie to get me out.

Sample 595. **Value 183.** Artificial sample.

My Favorite Book.

the book I refer to read is Ichabod Crane, it is an grate book and I like to rede it. Ichabod Crame was a man and a man wrote a book and it is called Ichabod Crane i like it because the man called it ichabod crane when I read it for it is such a great book.

Sample 618. **Value 260.** Artificial sample.

The Advantage of Tyranny.

Advantage evils are things of tyranny and there are many advantage evils. One thing is that when they opress the people they suffer awful I think it is a terrible thing when they say that you can be hanged down or trodden down without mercy and the tyranny does what they want there was tyrans in the revolutionary war and so they throwed off the yok.

Sample 94. **Value 369.** Written by a boy in the second year of the high school, aged 14 years.

Sulla as a Tyrant.

When Sulla came back from his conquest Marius had put himself consul so sulla with the army he had with him in his conquest siezed the government from Marius and put himself in consul and had a list of his enemys printy and the men whoes names were on this list we beheaded.

Hillegas, M.B. A scale for the measurement of quality in English composition by young people. Teachers College, Columbia University, 1912.

Figure 6.5   Thorndike Variable Maps (English composition, arithmetic, and language).

B. Arithmetic

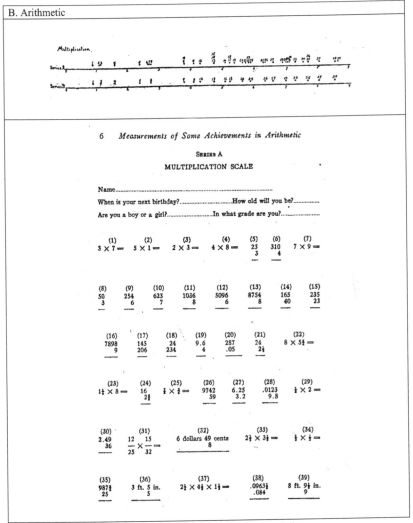

Woody, C. Measurements of some achievements in arithmetic. Teachers College,
Columbia University, 1920.

Figure 6.5   (Continued) Thorndike Variable Maps (English composition, arithmetic,
and language).

C. Completion -Test Language Scales

FIG. 2. Linear Projection of the Difficulty of the Sentences of Language Scale A.

Language Scale A   5

2. SCALE A, ITSELF

On each line of dots, write the word which makes the best meaning

ONLY ONE WORD ON EACH BLANK

II

x. The sky .... blue.
y. We are going .... school.

III

x. The kind lady .... the poor man a dollar.
y. The .... plays .... her dolls all day.

IV

x. Time .... often more valuable .... money.
y. Boys and .... soon become .... and women.

V

x. The poor baby .... as if it were .... sick.
y. The .... rises .... the morning and .... at night.

VI

x. It is good to hear .... voice .... friend.
y. She .... if she will.

VII

x. The poor little .... has .... nothing to ....; he is hungry.
y. The boy who .... hard .... do well.

VIII

x. Men .... more .... to do heavy work .... women.
y. It is a .... task to be kind to every beggar .... for money.

IX

x. Worry .... never improved a situation but has .... made conditions ....
y. A home is .... merely a place .... one .... live comfortably.

X

x. It is very .... to become .... acquainted .... persons who .... timid.
y. To .... many things .... ever finishing any of them .... a .... habit.

XI

x. One's real .... appears .... often in his .... than in his speech.
y. When one feels drowsy and ...., it .... happens that he is .... to fix his attention very successfully .... anything.

XII

x. The knowledge of .... use fire is .... of .... important things known by .... but unknown .... animals.
y. .... that are .... to one by an .... friend should be pardoned .... readily than injuries done by one .... is not angry.

XIII

x. To .... friends is always .... the .... it takes.
y. One ought to .... great care to .... the right .... of .... for one who .... bad habits .... it .... to get away from them.

Trabue, M.R. Completion -Test Language Scales. Teachers College, Columbia University, 1916.

Figure 6.5   (Continued) Thorndike Variable Maps (English composition, arithmetic, and language).

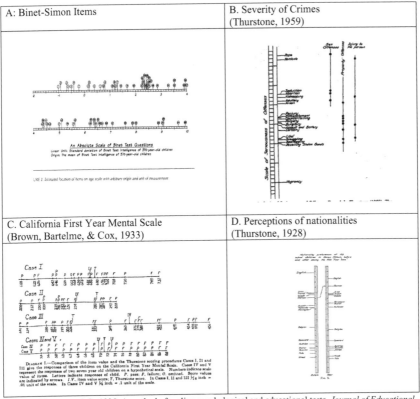

| A: Binet-Simon Items | B. Severity of Crimes (Thurstone, 1959) |
| C. California First Year Mental Scale (Brown, Bartelme, & Cox, 1933) | D. Perceptions of nationalities (Thurstone, 1928) |

A: Thurstone, L.L. 1925. A method of scaling psychological and educational tests. *Journal of Educational Psychology, 16,* 433– 451.

B: Thurstone, L.L. *The measurement of values.* The University of Chicago Press, 1959.

C: Brown, C. W. Bartelme, P. & Cox, G.M., 1933. The Scoring of individual performance on tests scaled according to the theory of absolute scaling. *Journal of Educational Psychology, 24*(9).

D: Thurstone, L. L. Experimental Study of Nationality Preferences. *Journal of General Psychology,* July -October, 1928.

Figure 6.6   Thurstone Variable Maps.

a set of Thurstone variable maps that include the mapping of Binet-Simon items (Panel A), perceived severity of various crimes (Panel B), California First Year Mental Scale (Panel, C), and perceptions of nationalities (Panel D). Panel B is interesting because it illustrates how Thurstone grouped item locations to highlight how perceptions of crime severity relates to sex offenses, property offenses, and personal injuries in a simple visual display. In Panel D, Thurstone (1928) uses a variable map to display how the perceptions of nationalities changed after viewing a movie. This display shows how the view of Germans changed over time.

Figure 6.7 provides a brief comparison between Birnbaum and Rasch item response functions with their implications for creating variable maps. Panel A in Figure 6.7 shows the Birnbaum items with intersecting item response functions (IRFs). Panel C shows the consequences of these crossing IRFs: there is no single variable map that unambiguously represents the locations of items that are invariant over person locations on the latent variable. Panel B, on the other hand, shows Rasch item response functions that do not intersect. Panel D illustrates that Rasch items yield invariant item locations across person locations. Wright (1997) clearly demonstrated how crossing item response functions imply that items have different locations on the variable map as a function of the location of the persons responding to the items.

An early Rasch variable map is given for the Knox Cube Test (Wright & Stone, 1979). Bond and Fox (2007) give a variable map for the BLOT test developed, while Engelhard and Myford (2003) show the variable map for AP English Literature and Composition. Other examples of variable maps include the Lexile Framework for Reading, and the Quantile Framework for Mathematics. Stone, Wright and Stenner (1999) provide a useful discussion of the historical origins of mapping, as well as a description of how variable maps can be used to conceptualize, develop, calibrate, monitor and revise our measures.

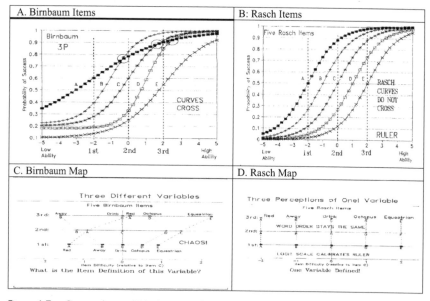

Figure 6.7   Comparison of Birnbaum and Rasch maps.

Discussion and Summary

This chapter focused on the quest for invariant measurement as illustrated by the research of selected measurement theorists working within the scaling tradition. This chapter builds on a series of earlier articles that I have written since the early 1980s describing invariant measurement from an historical perspective (Engelhard, 1984, 1991, 1992, 1994b, 2008a). As pointed out within the previous chapter, I view measurement theories in terms of two broad research traditions: test score tradition and scaling tradition. These traditions reflect paradigms that guide research workers in each area. The scaling tradition discussed in this chapter is emerging as the dominant paradigm for measurement in the 21st century. The theorists examined in this section made major contributions to our views of measurement in the scaling tradition. In discussing these measurement theorists, it is important to keep in mind the distinctions between parametric and nonparametric models, the concept of ideal-type models, the duality between person measurement and item calibration, and the key role of variable maps in measurement within the social, behavioral, and health sciences.

My intention in this chapter has been to delineate some of the central issues in invariant measurement, and to briefly examine how a selected group of measurement theories operating within the scaling traditions perceived these issues. The reader should be reminded of the limitations of any such list of issues. First of all, the measurement theorists may have changed their perspectives over time. Second, it is hard at times to infer from published work what the theorists may have actually thought about these issues. The goal is to provide starting points for further discussions of these issues, and to continue the illumination of some of the differences and similarities between the measurement models discussed in this chapter and the previous one. There is still much room for further discussion and debate regarding these issues. A final limitation is that variable maps inevitably present a simplified representation of a complex and multidimensional construct in two-dimensions (Monmonmier, 1996). It is argued that these simplifications as represented by variable maps still provide useful interpretive information. A detailed description for creating variable maps from a Rasch perspective is presented in Chapter 4.

Part III

Technical Issues

Chapter 7

Methods of Estimation for the Dichotomous Rasch Model

The focus of this chapter is on selected methods of estimation that have been proposed for Rasch models. Chapter 3 described an ideal-type view of measurement based on Rasch models that can yield invariant measurements. The next step in applying these measurement models is to estimate the Rasch model parameters that represent the locations of both items and persons on a variable map. The variable map provides an operational definition of the latent variable. Estimation is a key aspect of the measurement process that reflects the statistical problem of estimating model parameters within the context of an observed data set. Linacre (2004a, b) provides an overview of the major estimation methods used for estimating the parameters of Rasch measurement models. The basic underlying question addressed in this chapter is: How can we estimate the parameters (item and person location) of Rasch measurement models with real data?

After obtaining estimates of item and person locations on the latent variable by one of the methods described in this chapter, the next step is to examine the fit between the measurement model and observed data. Evaluation of model-data fit provides evidence regarding whether or not the requirements of invariant measurement have been approximated empirically by the data set in hand. Model-data fits issues related to Rasch measurement models are addressed in Chapter 8.

The first section of this chapter reviews the Dichotomous Model for Rasch measurement. Next, the general problem of estimation for measurement models is discussed, and specific estimation methods used for Rasch measurement models are identified. Following this section, the most common estimation methods used with the Dichotomous Model are described (non-iterative and iterative methods). The next section provides empirical examples of selected estimation methods using the learning stimulation scale from the HOME instrument described earlier (Monsaas & Engelhard, 1996). Finally, the main points of this chapter are discussed and summarized.

Dichotomous Model for Rasch Measurement

The Dichotomous Model is suitable for data collected with dichotomous scores or ratings (x = 0, 1) with two facets (persons and items). In this situation, the measurement problem is how to represent the observed data with estimated parameters that reflect the locations of persons and items on the latent variable. The operating characteristic (OC) function for the Dichotomous Model can be written as:

$$\phi_{ni1} = \frac{\exp(\theta_n - \delta_i)}{1 + \exp(\theta_n - \delta_i)} \qquad [1]$$

Equation 1 represents the conditional probability of person n (θ_n) on item i (δ_i) responding with a correct or positive response (x = 1). The differences between person and item locations on the line govern the probability of observing a incorrect/negative response (x = 0) or correct/positive response (x = 1). In essence, the statistical problem is to estimate the row and column values for persons and items that can be used to reproduce the observed responses in a data matrix.

Equation 1 can be used to represent the person response function for an individual (Person A) as follows:

$$Pr(x_{Ai} = 1|\theta_A, \delta_i) = \exp(\theta_A - \delta_i)/ [1 + \exp(\theta_A - \delta_i)] \qquad [2]$$

Equation 2 can also be shown graphically:

Person A

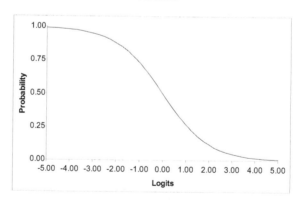

Equation 1 can also be used to represent the item response function for an item (Item 1):

$$Pr(x_{n1} = 1|\theta_n, \delta_1) = \exp(\theta_n - \delta_1)/ [1 + \exp(\theta_n - \delta_1)] \qquad [3]$$

The figure below provides a visual representation of Equation 3:

Item 1

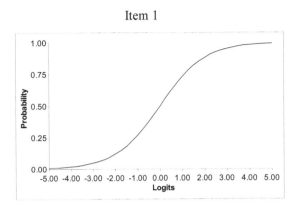

There are several things to remember before describing specific estimation methods. First of all, the θ-values and δ-values represent the locations of persons and items on the latent variable (variable map), respectively. It is also important to keep in mind the structure of observed data matrix with dichotomous data (x = 0, 1). The goal is to estimate row and column values (person and item locations) that can be used to represent the observed data matrix. The expected values for the cell entries are based on the Dichotomous Model. In other words, estimates of person and item locations can be inserted into the model to obtained expected values for entries in the data matrix. Finally, close fit between observed data and the expected values based on the model is needed to support the inference that invariant measurement has been obtained from the perspective of Rasch measurement.

It is important to recognize that the observed data can be conceptualized as follows:

Observed data = Expected values + Residuals

with Observed data (X = 0,1), Expected values obtained from inserting estimates in the model in Equation 1 (.00 > E > 1.00), and Residuals (−1.00 > R > 1.00) defined as follows:

Residuals = Observed data − Expected values.

Residuals can be used for quality control by aiding in the diagnosis of sources of model-data misfit. Methods for examining model-data fit are explored in Chapter 8.

For example, the edited data matrix for the Learning Stimulation Scale is presented in Table 7.1, which shows an edited version of the data matrix described in an earlier chapter with the rows sorted by person scores (low to high) and the columns sorted by item scores (easy to hard). One of the

Table 7.1   Observed Data: Learning Stimulation Scale (sorted and edited data with 37 persons and 11 items)

Person Score	Items: Person IDs	Items											Prop. correct score	Person Measures	SEM
		11 Easy	4	1	6	7	8	5	2	9	3	10 Hard			
High															
10	6	1	1	1	1	1	1	1	1	1	0	1	0.91	3.21	1.10
10	8	1	1	1	1	1	0	1	1	1	1	1	0.91	3.21	1.10
10	27	1	1	1	1	1	1	1	1	0	1	1	0.91	3.21	1.10
10	34	1	1	1	1	1	1	1	1	1	0	1	0.91	3.21	1.10
10	39	1	1	1	1	1	1	1	1	1	1	0	0.91	3.21	1.10
9	4	1	1	1	1	1	1	1	0	0	1	1	0.82	2.27	0.87
9	15	1	1	1	1	1	1	1	1	0	1	0	0.82	2.27	0.87
9	25	1	1	1	1	1	1	1	1	0	0	1	0.82	2.27	0.87
9	29	1	1	1	1	1	1	1	1	0	1	0	0.82	2.27	0.87
9	31	1	1	1	1	1	1	1	1	1	0	0	0.82	2.27	0.87
8	3	1	1	1	1	1	1	1	1	0	0	0	0.73	1.59	0.79
8	23	1	1	1	1	1	1	0	0	0	1	1	0.73	1.59	0.79
8	40	1	1	1	0	1	1	1	1	1	0	0	0.73	1.59	0.79
7	2	1	1	1	1	0	1	1	0	1	0	0	0.64	0.99	0.77
7	5	1	1	1	1	1	0	0	0	0	1	1	0.64	0.99	0.77
7	10	1	1	1	1	1	1	1	0	0	0	0	0.64	0.99	0.77
7	11	1	1	1	1	1	1	0	1	0	0	0	0.64	0.99	0.77
7	12	1	1	1	1	1	1	1	0	0	0	0	0.64	0.99	0.77
7	18	1	1	1	1	1	0	0	1	1	0	0	0.64	0.99	0.77

Score	Item	35	34	32	30	24	22	21	16	14	12	10	P-value	Item Location	Item SEM
7	22	1	1	0	1	1	1	0	0	1	1	0	0.64	0.99	0.77
7	30	1	1	1	1	1	0	0	1	1	0	0	0.64	0.99	0.77
7	38	1	1	1	1	1	1	1	0	0	0	1	0.64	0.99	0.77
6	13	1	1	1	1	0	1	0	0	0	1	0	0.55	0.41	0.77
6	14	1	1	1	1	0	1	0	0	0	1	0	0.55	0.41	0.77
6	17	1	1	1	1	0	0	1	1	0	0	0	0.55	0.41	0.77
6	24	1	1	0	1	0	1	1	0	1	0	0	0.55	0.41	0.77
6	32	1	1	1	1	1	0	1	0	0	0	0	0.55	0.41	0.77
6	35	1	1	1	1	0	1	0	0	0	0	1	0.55	0.41	0.77
6	37	1	1	1	1	0	0	1	1	0	0	0	0.55	0.41	0.77
5	16	1	1	1	1	0	0	0	1	0	0	0	0.45	-0.19	0.79
5	20	1	1	1	1	0	1	0	0	0	0	0	0.45	-0.19	0.79
4	21	1	1	1	0	0	0	1	0	0	0	0	0.36	-0.83	0.82
3	7	0	1	1	0	0	0	0	1	0	0	0	0.27	-1.53	0.87
3	26	1	0	0	0	1	0	0	0	1	0	0	0.27	-1.53	0.87
2	19	1	0	0	1	0	0	0	0	0	0	0	0.18	-2.34	0.94
2	33	1	1	0	0	0	0	0	0	0	0	0	0.18	-2.34	0.94
2	36	0	0	1	1	0	0	0	0	0	0	0	0.18	-2.34	0.94
Low	Item Score:	35	34	32	30	24	22	21	16	14	12	10			
	P-value:	0.95	0.92	0.86	0.81	0.65	0.59	0.57	0.43	0.38	0.32	0.27			
	Item Location:	-3.01	-2.47	-1.71	-1.14	0.08	0.41	0.57	1.33	1.64	1.97	2.32			
	Item SEM:	.79	.68	.57	.50	.41	.40	.40	.39	.40	.41	.43			

Note. Rasch item locations and person measures are obtained from the JMLE Method using the Facets computer program.

preliminary steps for examining data is to sort data matrix using person and item scores. This simple process highlights missing data, and facilitates the removal of response vectors with all zeros or ones. In these data, three pre-school children have home environments with all of the items present (Persons 1, 9, and 28), and these are not included in Table 7.1. Perfect response patterns with all items present or absent are not included in the estimation process, although it is possible to impute values for these children. For persons, the proportion correct scores range from Person 6 who lives in a highly stimulating learning environment with 10 out of the 11 items present (Proportion correct score of .91) to Person 36 who lives in a less stimulating environment with only 2 items present (Items 1 and 6).

Rasch person and item locations (measures) with standard errors of measurement (SEM) are included in Table 7.1. These person and item estimates were obtained based on the Joint Maximum Likelihood (JMLE) Method using the Facets computer program (Linacre, 2007). The JMLE Method is described later in this chapter. Based on these estimated values, it is possible to obtain the expected ratings for each person and item. Since scores are sufficient statistics for estimating person locations, each person with the same score has the same location on the variable map (person measure).

Table 7.2 shows the expected responses by person score and item difficulty. Columns 1 to 4 present the person scores, frequency of persons with that score, proportion correct score, and person measures (locations). Columns 5 to 15 show the expected responses based on the model. There are several things to note in Table 7.2. First of all, the probability of correct responses increases across rows for Item 1 (easy item) to Item 10 (hard item) as expected. Secondly, the probabilities decrease down the columns as person scores go from a score of 10 (high score) to 2 (low score). The reader should note that this reflects a probabilistic Guttman pattern.

Table 7.3 presents the observed, expected and residual scores for two persons. These two persons have the same scores on the learning stimulation scale (Person scores = 6). The first column in this table lists the items from easy to hard. The next four columns report the observed (O), expected (E), residual (R), and absolute value of residual (|R|) scores for Person 17. Comparable values are presented for Person 24. The last column provides the item labels. Person 17 has a good fit or correspondence between the observed and expected scores with the sum of the absolute values of the residuals fairly small (|R| = 2.64). Person 24 has a poorer fit between the observed and expected responses (|R| = 5.42). Even though both persons have the same score and estimated location on the latent variable, it is clear that the total score does not reflect the same home environments for both of these persons. For example, Person 17 does not have magazines, a music player, newspaper or puzzles, while Person 24 with the same score of 6 has a music player and newspapers in the home environment.

The next chapter presents methods for exploring model-data fit in more detail based on the residuals defined as the differences between observed and expected responses obtained after estimating person and item parameters.

Table 7.2 Expected responses by person scores and item difficulty: Joint Maximum Likelihood Estimation Method

Person Score	Freq.	Prop. correct	Person Measure	Easy				Items						Hard
				11	4	1	6	7	8	5	2	9	3	10
				-3.01	-2.47	-1.71	-1.14	0.08	0.41	0.57	1.33	1.64	1.97	2.32
High														
10	5	0.91	3.21	1.00	1.00	0.99	0.99	0.96	0.94	0.93	0.87	0.83	0.78	0.71
9	5	0.82	2.27	0.99	0.99	0.98	0.97	0.90	0.87	0.85	0.72	0.65	0.57	0.49
8	3	0.64	1.59	0.99	0.98	0.96	0.94	0.82	0.76	0.74	0.56	0.49	0.41	0.33
7	9	0.64	0.99	0.98	0.97	0.94	0.89	0.71	0.64	0.60	0.41	0.34	0.27	0.21
6	7	0.55	0.41	0.97	0.95	0.89	0.82	0.58	0.50	0.46	0.28	0.23	0.17	0.13
5	2	0.45	-0.19	0.94	0.91	0.82	0.72	0.43	0.35	0.32	0.18	0.14	0.10	0.08
4	1	0.36	-0.83	0.90	0.84	0.71	0.58	0.29	0.22	0.20	0.10	0.08	0.06	0.04
3	2	0.27	-1.53	0.81	0.72	0.54	0.40	0.17	0.13	0.11	0.05	0.04	0.03	0.02
2	3	0.18	-2.34	0.66	0.53	0.35	0.23	0.08	0.06	0.05	0.02	0.02	0.01	0.01
Low	N = 37													

Note. Person scores (sum of correct or positive responses) are sufficient statistics for estimating person measures (locations), and therefore persons with the same scores can be grouped together.

Table 7.3 Responses for Persons 17 (Good model-data fit) and 24 (Poor model-data fit) on the Learning Stimulation Scale (both with observed scores of 6): JMLE Method

Item	Person 17: Good Fit				Person 24: Poor Fit				Item Label
	O	E	R	$|R|$	O	E	R	$|R|$	
Hard									
10	0	0.13	-0.13	0.13	0	0.13	-0.13	0.13	Magazines
3	0	0.17	-0.17	0.17	1	0.17	0.83	0.83	Music player
9	0	0.23	-0.23	0.23	1	0.23	0.77	0.77	Newspapers
2	0	0.28	-0.28	0.28	0	0.28	-0.28	0.28	Puzzles
5	1	0.46	0.54	0.54	1	0.46	0.54	0.54	Toys (Refined movements)
8	0	0.50	-0.50	0.50	1	0.50	0.50	0.50	Ten books visible
7	1	0.58	0.42	0.42	0	0.58	-0.58	0.58	Ten or more children's books
6	1	0.82	0.18	0.18	0	0.82	-0.82	0.82	Toys (Teach numbers)
1	1	0.89	0.11	0.11	0	0.89	-0.89	0.89	Toys (Color size and shape)
4	1	0.95	0.05	0.05	1	0.95	0.05	0.05	Toys (Free expression)
11	1	0.97	0.03	0.03	1	0.97	0.03	0.03	Shapes
Easy									
Sum	6	5.98	0.02	2.64	6	5.98	0.02	5.42	

Note. Both persons have the same score and location on the latent variable. O is the observed score, E is the expected score, R is the residual score, and |R| is the absolute value of the residual that can be used to examine fit.

Methods of Estimation

In order to put a measurement model to work, methods for estimating its parameters from suitable data must be developed.

(Wright, 1980, p. 188)

Estimation is a basic statistical and mathematical process that addresses how to obtain estimates for parameters in models. The major approaches for obtaining estimates include least squares, maximum likelihood (Fisher, 1922, 1925), Bayesian approaches (Swaminathan & Gifford, 1982), and non-parametric and data intensive methods including Functional Data Analysis (Ramsey & Silverman, 2002). It is beyond the scope of this text to address each of these estimation methods in detail. Each estimation method has strengths and weaknesses, and the interested and motivated reader should seek out the original sources and presentations of each of the estimation methods. The key point for researchers is that point estimates of person and item locations within the context of Rasch measurement obtained from different estimation methods are usually indistinguishable from one another. However, the standard errors that quantify the uncertainty in these estimates can vary significantly by estimation method. This variation is based on the underlying assumptions of each estimation method. Of course, this is one of the very tricky issues in statistics: How can we quantify uncertainty in our parameter estimates?

Within the context of Rasch measurement, there is another estimation issue that should be considered. In most applications, there is an asymmetry in estimates of person locations as compared to item locations. Typically, item locations are estimated more precisely than the person locations because the item locations are based on many persons having taken that items, while person location estimates are usually based on that person having taken only a limited number of items. As pointed out by Rasch (1960/1980):

In practice, therefore, the parameters for persons and for items enter into the problem in a quite asymmetric way: *few degrees of difficulty estimated with great certainty, and many degrees of ability each estimated rather poorly.* [italics in the original] (p. 77).

Estimation methods for Rasch models can be categorized as non-iterative and iterative. Non-iterative methods involve estimation equations that can be solved in closed form. Iterative methods are based on the principle of maximum likelihood, and they require numerical methods, such as Newton-Raphson, with multiple steps to solve the likelihood equations. In essence, iterative processes are defined as numerical methods that involve providing an initial guess or estimate (starting value) for an unknown value that provides a solution to an equation, and the repeated correction of these guesses in order to obtain better estimates of these unknown values. The repeated corrections are called iterations, and these iterations continue until an acceptable stopping criterion is provided. For example, Newton-Raphson is a common iterative process that can be used to obtain item and person locations as shown later in this chapter. The non-iterative methods are the LOG Method, the PAIR Method, and the PROX Method. The iterative methods are JMLE Method, MML Method, and CML Method.

Non-Iterative Estimation Methods

I. LOG Method

LOG is easy to follow and brings out in an especially clear way the decisive part that additivity plays in the construction of a measuring system.

(Wright, 1980, p. 188)

Rasch (1960/1980) described the LOG method as a simple way to fit a two-way linear model without interactions to item and score groups. This method highlights the simple additive structure of the Dichotomous Model. It also provides for the opportunity to create graphical displays that highlight aspects of invariant measurement. The LOG Method is a non-iterative method based on the principle of least squares.

The basic steps for the LOG Method are as follows:

1. Create score groups (raw-score groups)
2. Calculate logs of the ratios of item successes to failures within each score group
3. Fit a two-way linear model with no interactions
4. Plot the data to examine model-data fit

The LOG Method illustrates the underlying notion of invariant measurement in a very intuitive way for researchers. The LOG Method has didactic value, but it is not currently used as an operational estimation method for Rasch models.

2. PAIR Method

It is my opinion that only through systematic comparisons—experimental or observational—is possible to formulate empirical laws of sufficient generalizability to be—speaking frankly—of real value.

(Rasch, 1977, pp. 68–69)

Rasch (1960/1980) suggested another non-iterative method of estimation based on the principle of paired comparisons. Rasch (1960/1980) described a PAIR Method for estimating the item parameters in the Dichotomous Model that was suggested by Gustav Leunbach with the person parameters completely removed by conditioning (Wright, 1980). The underlying idea of using pairwise comparisons can be traced back to work by Fechner (1860) in psychophysics. Thurstone (1927) used the method of paired comparisons to scale attitudes and values. This method provides a clear framework for item calibration, and the development of item banks. Choppin (1968) highlighted the use of the PAIR Method for data sets with missing data.

In essence, the PAIR Method models differences in the locations between two items with the person parameter cancelling out of the equation. The PAIR Method has been described in detail by Choppin (1985). Andrich (1988) provides another nice description of the PAIR Method. Recently, Mary Garner has advanced our appreciation for the PAIR Method by highlighting its connection to well-known numerical methods based on estimating eigenvalues and eigenvectors of pairwise and adjacency matrices (Garner, 1998; Garner & Engelhard, 2000, 2002). The Eigenvector Method has been used to obtained estimates of Rasch parameters for dichotomous and polytomous data (Garner & Engelhard, 2010), and it has also been extended to address issues related rater-mediated assessments (Garner & Engelhard, 2009).

Following Garner and Engelhard (2000), the basic steps for the PAIR Method are as follows:

1. Create a paired comparison matrix (item by item comparisons)
2. Entries above the diagonal indicate count of persons who succeed on the first item and fail on the second item in the pairs
3. Fit a linear model to logs of cell entries (least squares, maximum likelihood, EV method)

The various pairwise estimation methods focus on item calibrations with person measurement viewed as a separate step. There are advantages and disadvantages to this approach. Pairwise algorithms are very useful for item banking with incomplete and missing data (Choppin, 1985), and also for test equating to create vertical scales (Engelhard & Osberg, 1983). The PAIR Method is currently used in the RUMM software (Andrich, Lyne, Sheridan, & Luo, 2000).

3. PROX Method

Cohen (1979) has suggested a non-iterative method based on the assumption that item and person locations are normally distributed. His PROX Method is simple, and the calculations can easily be done by hand or with a spreadsheet program, such as Excel. An iterative version has been developed by Linacre (2007b), and it is currently used to provide starting values for the JMLE Method in several computer programs, such as Winsteps and Facets.

The basic steps for the non-iterative PROX Method are presented in Table 7.4. The first column in Table 7.4 lists the steps for the PROX Method of estimation. The second column summarizes the essential equations, and the last column describes the steps. Steps 1 to 4 provide preliminary person logits (Panel A), Steps 5 to 8 provide the preliminary item logits (Panel B), Panel C shows the adjustments necessary for obtaining invariance for item locations (Step 9) and for person locations (Step 10), and finally, Steps 11 and 12 (Panel

Table 7.4   Steps in the Estimation of Person and Item Locations with PROX Method (Cohen, 1979)

Step	Equations	Description
Panel A: Preliminary Person Logits		
1	$$p_i = \sum_{j=1}^{L} x_{ij} / L$$	Mean of person-correct scores [$p_i \equiv$ proportion-correct score for person i, L is the number of items]
2	$$\hat{\theta}_{i1} = \ln[p_i/(1-p_i)]$$	Preliminary estimates of person logits
3	$$\overline{\theta} = \sum_{i=1}^{N} \hat{\theta}_i / N$$	Mean of person logits
4	$$\hat{\sigma}_{\hat{\theta}}^2 = \sum_{i=1}^{N} (\hat{\theta}_{i1} - \overline{\theta})^2 / (N-1)$$	Variance of person logits
Panel B: Preliminary Item Logits		
5	$$p_j = \sum_{i=1}^{N} x_{ij} / N$$	Mean of item-correct scores [$p_j \equiv$ p-value for item j, N is the number of persons]
6	$$\hat{\delta}_{j1} = \ln[(1-p_j)/p_j]$$	Preliminary estimates of item logits
7	$$\overline{\delta} = \sum_{j=1}^{L} \hat{\delta}_j / L$$	Mean of item logits
8	$$\hat{\sigma}_{\hat{\delta}}^2 = \sum_{j=1}^{L} (\hat{\delta}_j - \overline{\delta})^2 / L - 1$$	Variance of item logits
Panel C: Adjustments for invariance		
9	$$A_{items} = \left(\frac{1 + \hat{\sigma}_{\hat{\delta}}^2 / 2.89}{1 + \hat{\sigma}_{\hat{\delta}}^2 \hat{\sigma}_{\hat{\theta}}^2 / 8.35)} \right)^{1/2}$$	Adjustment for variation in items
10	$$A_{persons} = \left(\frac{1 + \hat{\sigma}_{\hat{\theta}}^2 / 2.89}{1 + \hat{\sigma}_{\hat{\delta}}^2 \hat{\sigma}_{\hat{\theta}}^2 / 8.35)} \right)^{1/2}$$	Adjustment for variation in persons
Panel D: PROX Estimates of person and item locations		
11	$$\hat{\theta}_{i2} = A_{items}\left[\hat{\theta}_{i1}\right]$$	PROX estimates of person locations
12	$$\hat{\delta}_{j2} = A_{persons}\left[\hat{\delta}_{j1} - \overline{\delta}\right]$$	PROX estimates of item locations: centered logits (subtract mean of items)

D) provide the final equations for obtaining the estimates of person and item locations based on the PROX Method.

4. Illustrative Data Analyses for Non-Iterative Methods of Estimation

This section illustrates the use of several methods for estimating the parameters of the Dichotomous Models using the three non-iterative methods of estimation: LOG, PAIR, and PROX Methods. In each of the estimation methods, preliminary steps include the sorting the data matrix by person and item scores. This sorted matrix can provide a useful first step for visualizing patterns in the data set. This sorted data matrix has been called a Scalogram within the context of Guttman scaling (Engelhard, 2005). Next, perfect person and item response patterns are dropped from the data set. The rationale is that locations for persons who answer all of the items incorrectly or correctly were not targeted appropriately (items were either too hard or too easy for the persons), and therefore do not provide useful measurement information. Locations can be assigned to persons with perfect response patterns, but they cannot be directly estimated from the observed data set. A similar rationale justifies the elimination of items that are answered incorrectly or correctly by all of the persons.

The LOG Method is illustrated first. The data in Table 7.1 have been sorted with perfect person and item response patterns deleted. The total number of persons is now 37. Panel A in Table 7.5 presents these data grouped by scores and Panel B shows the proportion correct in each cell. For example, there were 3 persons with a score of 2, and 2 out of 3 persons (.667) answered Item 11 correctly. The bottom panel gives the log of the ratios of item successes to failures within each score group. Perfect proportions of (0.00) and (1.00) in Panel B are replaced with 0.05 and 0.95 respectively for the calculation of the logits shown in Panel C. This is done because logs cannot be obtained for these proportions (Bock & Jones, 1968). In larger data sets, these extreme values would not be as frequently observed. For example, score 2 for Item 1 with a proportion correct of .667 yields a value of $-.693$ logits: Ln $[(1 - .667)/ .667]$. Next, the row and column means are calculated for these data (two-way linear model with no interactions). The LOG item measures are obtained by calculating the weighted mean for each item over score groups.

The next estimation method illustrated in this section is the Pair Method. Table 7.6 presents an illustration of the use of the PAIR Method for the first four items from the Learning Stimulation Scale. Panel A gives the inequalities that are used to construct the comparisons for the pairs of items. Panel B provides the count matrix (C-matrix) for Items 1 to 4: the number of times that the response to items pairs were answered correctly on an item compared to another item. Panel C gives the proportions, while Panel C presents the logits for these proportions. The means of these logits provide estimates of the item locations.

Table 7.5 Illustration of the LOG Method (Learning Stimulation Scale)

Score	Freq.	Easy					Items										Hard
		11	4	32	1	30	7	22	21	5	2	16	14	9	12	3	10
Panel A: Responses grouped by total scores																	
High 10	5	5	5	5	5	5	5	4	5	5	5	5	4	4	3	3	4
9	5	5	5	5	5	5	5	5	5	5	4	4	1	1	3	3	2
8	3	3	3	3	3	2	3	3	2	2	2	2	1	1	1	1	1
7	9	9	9	8	8	8	8	5	4	4	3	3	5	5	2	2	2
6	7	7	7	6	6	6	2	4	4	4	1	1	1	1	3	3	1
5	2	2	2	2	2	2	0	1	0	0	0	0	1	1	0	0	0
4	1	1	1	1	1	1	0	0	1	1	0	0	0	0	0	0	0
3	2	1	1	1	1	0	1	0	0	0	1	1	1	1	0	0	0
Low 2	3	2	1	1	1	1	0	0	0	0	0	0	0	0	0	0	0
Item																	
Sum	N=37	35	34	32	32	30	24	22	21	21	16	16	14	14	12	12	10
Panel B: Percentages																	
High 10	5	(1.00)	(1.00)	(1.00)	(1.00)	(1.00)	(1.00)	0.800	(1.00)	(1.00)	(1.00)	(1.00)	0.800	0.800	0.600	0.600	0.800
9	5	(1.00)	(1.00)	(1.00)	(1.00)	(1.00)	(1.00)	(1.00)	(1.00)	(1.00)	0.800	0.800	0.200	0.200	0.600	0.600	0.400
8	3	(1.00)	(1.00)	(1.00)	(1.00)	0.667	(1.00)	(1.00)	0.667	0.667	0.667	0.667	0.333	0.333	0.333	0.333	0.333
7	9	(1.00)	(1.00)	0.889	0.889	0.889	0.889	0.556	0.444	0.444	0.333	0.333	0.556	0.556	0.222	0.222	0.222
6	7	(1.00)	(1.00)	0.857	0.857	0.857	0.286	0.571	0.571	0.571	0.143	0.143	0.143	0.143	0.429	0.429	0.143

5	2	(1.00)	(1.00)	(1.00)	(1.00)	(0.00)	0.500	(0.00)	(0.00)	0.500	(0.00)	(0.00)
4	1	(1.00)	(1.00)	(1.00)	(0.00)	(0.00)	(0.00)	(1.00)	0.500	(0.00)	(0.00)	(0.00)
3	2	0.500	0.500	0.500	(0.00)	0.500	(0.00)	(0.00)	(0.00)	0.500	(0.00)	(0.00)
Low 2	3	0.667	0.333	0.667	0.667	(0.00)	0.500	(0.00)	(0.00)	(0.00)	(0.00)	(0.00)

Panel C: Item Logits

High 10	5	-2.944	-2.944	-2.944	-2.944	-2.944	-1.386	-2.944	-2.944	-1.386	-0.405	-1.386
9	5	-2.944	-2.944	-2.944	-2.944	-2.944	-2.944	-2.944	-1.386	1.386	-0.405	0.405
8	3	-2.944	-2.944	-0.693	-0.693	-2.944	-2.944	-0.693	-0.693	0.693	0.693	0.693
7	9	-2.944	-2.944	-2.079	-2.079	-2.079	-0.223	0.223	0.693	-0.223	1.253	1.253
6	7	-2.944	-2.944	-1.792	-1.792	0.916	-0.288	-0.288	1.792	1.792	0.288	1.792
5	2	-2.944	-2.944	-2.944	-2.944	2.944	0.000	2.944	2.944	0.000	2.944	2.944
4	1	-2.944	-2.944	-2.944	2.944	2.944	2.944	-2.944	2.944	2.944	2.944	2.944
3	2	0.000	0.000	0.000	2.944	0.000	2.944	2.944	0.000	0.000	2.944	2.944
Low 2	3	-0.693	0.693	0.693	-0.693	2.944	2.944	2.944	-0.693	2.944	2.944	2.944
Weighted Item Mean		-2.603	-2.490	-2.062	-1.673	-0.890	-0.455	-0.375	0.344	0.659	0.942	1.204

Note. Perfect proportions of (0.00) and (1.00) in Panel B are replaced with 0.05 and 0.95 respectively for the calculation of the logits in Panel C.

Table 7.6   Illustration of the PAIR Method (Items 1 to 4)

Person	I1	I2	I3	I4
2	1	0	0	1
3	1	1	0	1
4	1	0	1	1
5	1	0	1	1
6	1	1	0	1
7	1	1	0	1
8	1	1	1	1
10	1	0	0	1
11	1	1	0	1
12	1	0	0	1
13	1	0	1	1
14	1	0	1	1
15	1	1	1	1
16	1	0	0	1
17	1	0	0	1
18	1	1	0	1
19	0	0	0	0
20	1	0	0	1
21	1	0	0	1
22	0	0	1	1
23	1	0	1	1
24	0	0	1	1
25	1	1	0	1
26	0	0	0	0
27	1	1	1	1
29	1	1	1	1
30	1	1	0	1
31	1	1	0	1
32	1	0	0	1
33	0	0	0	1
34	1	1	0	1
35	1	0	0	1
36	1	0	0	0
37	1	1	0	1

Panel A: Comparisons

Items	I1	I2	I3	I4
I1	.	I1>I2	I1>I3	I1>I4
I2	I2>I1	.	I2>I3	I2>I4
I3	I3>I1	I3>I2	.	I3>I4
I4	I4>I1	I4>I2	I4>I3	.

Panel B: C Matrix (Item comparisons)

	I1	I2	I3	I4
I1	.	15	22	1
I2	0	.	12	0
I3	2	7	.	0
I4	3	17	22	.

Panel C: Proportions

	I1	I2	I3	I4
I1	.	(1.00)	0.917	0.250
I2	(0.00)	.	0.632	(0.00)
I3	0.083	0.368	.	(0.00)
I4	0.750	(1.00)	(1.00)	.

Panel D: Logits= ln [p/(1-p)]

	I1	I2	I3	I4
I1	.	2.944	2.398	-1.099
I2	-2.944	.	0.539	-2.944
I3	-2.398	-0.539	.	-2.944
I4	1.099	2.944	2.944	.
Item Difficulty	-1.414	0.802	0.981	-2.329

Person	I1	I2	I3	I4
38	1	0	0	1
39	1	1	1	1
40	1	1	0	1

Note. Perfect proportions of (0.00) and (1.00) in Panel B are replaced with 0.05 and 0.95 respectively for the calculation of the logits.

Table 7.6 describes in detail the calculation of the pairwise comparisons for Items 1 to 4 from the scale. The left side of the Table 7.7 presents the responses from the 37 persons for Items 1 to 4. The right side of the table illustrates the counting algorithm that is used to obtain the paired comparisons used to estimate item difficulties. Panel A describes the comparisons made to obtain the count matrix (C) that is shown in Panel B. For example, Item 1 has responses larger than Item 2 for 15 persons, and there are zero responses where Item 2 is larger than Item 1. Panel C gives the proportions that correspond to the counts in Panel B, while Panel D provides the logits transformation of these proportions. The final estimates of the item difficulties in logits are –1.414, 0.802, 0.981, and –2.329.

The PROX Method of estimation was described in Table 7.4. As pointed out earlier, the PROX Method essentially involves the calculation of person and item logits with adjustments to account for the sample dependence of these preliminary estimates of person and items locations.

The PROX estimates for the 11 items on the Learning Stimulation Scale are shown in Table 7.7.

Table 7.7   Illustration of PROX Method for Learning Stimulation Scale (Item measures, L=11)

Item	Item Sum	P-value	Item Logit	Centered Logit	Item Locations
11	35	0.95	-2.86	-2.19	-2.47
4	34	0.92	-2.43	-1.76	-1.99
1	32	0.86	-1.86	-1.19	-1.34
6	30	0.81	-1.46	-0.79	-0.89
7	24	0.65	-0.61	0.06	0.07
8	22	0.59	-0.38	0.29	0.33
5	21	0.57	-0.27	0.40	0.45
2	16	0.43	0.27	0.94	1.06
9	14	0.38	0.50	1.17	1.32
3	12	0.32	0.73	1.40	1.58
10	10	0.27	0.99	1.66	1.88
Mean			-0.67	-0.00	-0.00
Item Variance= 1.71					

Table 7.8   Illustration of PROX Method for Learning Stimulation Scale
(Person measures, N=37)

Person	Person Score	Proportion Correct	Person Logits	Person Locations
6	10	0.91	2.30	2.44
8	10	0.91	2.30	2.44
27	10	0.91	2.30	2.44
34	10	0.91	2.30	2.44
39	10	0.91	2.30	2.44
4	9	0.82	1.50	1.59
15	9	0.82	1.50	1.59
25	9	0.82	1.50	1.59
29	9	0.82	1.50	1.59
31	9	0.82	1.50	1.59
3	8	0.73	0.98	1.04
23	8	0.73	0.98	1.04
40	8	0.73	0.98	1.04
2	7	0.64	0.56	0.59
5	7	0.64	0.56	0.59
10	7	0.64	0.56	0.59
11	7	0.64	0.56	0.59
12	7	0.64	0.56	0.59
18	7	0.64	0.56	0.59
22	7	0.64	0.56	0.59
30	7	0.64	0.56	0.59
38	7	0.64	0.56	0.59
13	6	0.55	0.18	0.19
14	6	0.55	0.18	0.19
17	6	0.55	0.18	0.19
24	6	0.55	0.18	0.19
32	6	0.55	0.18	0.19
35	6	0.55	0.18	0.19
37	6	0.55	0.18	0.19
16	5	0.45	-0.18	-0.19
20	5	0.45	-0.18	-0.19
21	4	0.36	-0.56	-0.59
7	3	0.27	-0.98	-1.04
26	3	0.27	-0.98	-1.04
19	2	0.18	-1.50	-1.59
33	2	0.18	-1.50	-1.59
36	2	0.18	-1.50	-1.59

Mean   0.55
Person Variance =1.14

The person estimates are shown in Table 7.8. The adjustments to obtain invariant item calibrations and person measures for these data are shown below:

Adjustments for invariance (Steps 9 and 10)

Steps   **Equation**   **Observed data**

9

$$A_{items} = \left(\frac{1+\hat{\sigma}_{\delta}^2/2.89)}{1+\hat{\sigma}_{\delta}^2\hat{\sigma}_{\theta}^2/8.35)} \right)^{1/2} \quad A_{items} = \left(\frac{1+(1.71/2.89)}{1+(1.71\times1.14)/8.35} \right)^{1/2} = \sqrt{\frac{1.59}{1.23}} = 1.13$$

10

$$A_{persons} = \left(\frac{1+\hat{\sigma}_{\theta}^2/2.89)}{1+\hat{\sigma}_{\delta}^2\hat{\sigma}_{\theta}^2/8.35)} \right)^{1/2} \quad A_{persons} = \left(\frac{1+(1.14/2.89)}{1+(1.71\times1.14)/8.35} \right)^{1/2} = \sqrt{\frac{1.39}{1.23}} = 1.06$$

It should be noted that 2.89 (1.7^2) and 8.35 (2.89^2) are the constants used to bring the normal deviates from the normal distribution into line with the logits based on the logistic distribution (Wright & Stone, 1979).

Table 7.9 presents a comparison of three non-iterative methods for calibrating items (LOG, PAIR and PROX) with an iterative method—Joint Maximum Likelihood Estimation (JMLE) Method—that is used in the Facets program (Linacre, 2007). The item difficulties are comparable, but it should be noted that the units are slightly different for each method as reflected in the range of standard deviations (SD) from 1.38 to 1.83 logits. For the purposes of comparing the item calibrations, Table 7.10 was constructed with the item difficulties

Table 7.9   Comparison of Unstandardized Item Calibrations

Item Number	Item Score	P-value	LOG Method	PAIR Method	PROX Method	JMLE Method
10	10	0.27	1.20	2.23	1.88	2.32
3	12	0.32	0.94	1.74	1.58	1.97
9	14	0.38	0.66	1.43	1.32	1.64
2	16	0.43	0.34	1.30	1.06	1.33
5	21	0.57	-0.38	0.62	0.45	0.57
8	22	0.59	-0.46	0.53	0.33	0.41
7	24	0.65	-0.89	0.08	0.07	0.08
6	30	0.81	-1.67	-0.68	-0.89	-1.14
1	32	0.86	-2.06	-1.28	-1.34	-1.71
4	34	0.92	-2.49	-2.73	-1.99	-2.47
11	35	0.95	-2.60	-3.23	-2.47	-3.01
Mean			-0.67	0.00	0.00	0.00
SD			1.38	1.80	1.48	1.83

Note. Item calibrations for the PAIR Method are from Garner and Engelhard (2000)

Table 7.10 Comparison of Standardized Item Calibrations (Mean = .00, SD = 1.00)

Item Number	Item Score	P-value	LOG Method	PAIR Method	PROX Method	JMLE Method
10	10	0.27	1.36	1.24	1.27	1.27
3	12	0.32	1.17	0.97	1.07	1.08
9	14	0.38	0.96	0.79	0.89	0.90
2	16	0.43	0.73	0.72	0.72	0.73
5	21	0.57	0.21	0.34	0.30	0.31
8	22	0.59	0.15	0.29	0.22	0.22
7	24	0.65	-0.16	0.04	0.05	0.04
6	30	0.81	-0.72	-0.38	-0.60	-0.62
1	32	0.86	-1.01	-0.71	-0.91	-0.93
4	34	0.92	-1.32	-1.52	-1.34	-1.35
11	35	0.95	-1.40	-1.79	-1.67	-1.64
Mean			0.00	0.00	0.00	0.00
SD			1.00	1.00	1.00	1.00

from the four estimation methods centered on zero, and the standard deviations adjusted to have a value of one within each method. It is clear from Table 7.10 that the item calibrations are basically equivalent across the four estimation methods.

Iterative Estimation Methods

The previous section described three non-iterative estimation methods (LOG, PAIR, and PROX Methods), and this section describes three iterative estimation methods (JMLE, MML, and CML Methods). These three iterative methods are all based on the principles of maximum likelihood estimation developed by Fisher (1922, 1925).

Enders (2005) provides a clear description of the underlying principles of maximum likelihood (ML) Method. The ML Method is designed to obtain estimated parameter values (item and person locations for the Rasch models) that maximize the likelihood of obtaining the observed data based on the proposed measurement model. The concept of likelihood is related to the concept of probability. In essence, probabilities describe future events, while likelihoods address events that have already occurred and the researcher is determining what events made the observed outcomes the most likely. One of the advantages of ML estimation is that the second derivative of likelihood function is used in most numerical methods, and it provides an estimate of uncertainty that can be used to define standard errors for the parameter estimates.

I. JMLE Method

The most common method used to obtain parameter estimates for Rasch models is based on the Joint Maximum Likelihood Estimation (JMLE) Method. This method was described in detail by Wright & Panchapakesan (1969). It is sometimes called the UCON Method in the Rasch measurement literature. The JMLE Method is used in all of the major Rasch computer programs, such as Winsteps and Facets (Linacre, 2007).

In the 1950s, the sociologist Paul Lazarsfeld introduced the principle of local independence (Lazarsfeld, 1950) based on research conducted during World War II (Stouffer et al., 1950). Local independence is defined as the statistical independence of item responses when persons have the same location on the latent variable (Bock, 1977). If we assume that the responses of each person are independent given their location on the latent variable (θ), then the likelihood of observing a particular response vector for a person is

$$P(\theta) = \prod_{i=1}^{L} P_i^{x_i}(1 - P_i)^{1-x_i} \qquad [4]$$

where x_i represents the dichotomous response of the person to item i (0=incorrect, 1=correct), $P_i(\theta)$ represents the condition probability of succeeding on item i given the Rasch model, $\prod$ is the multiplication operator that indicates multiplication of each of the terms in the equation (i to L). In the case of the dichotomous Rasch model, the conditional probability is given as

$$Pr(x_{ni} = 1|\theta_n, \delta_i) = \exp(\theta_n - \delta_i)/ [1 + \exp(\theta_n - \delta_i)] \qquad [5]$$

Fisher (1922, 1925) has called Equation 4 the likelihood equation. If we assume that the item parameters in the Rasch model are known, then Equations 4 can be used to obtain maximum likelihood estimates of the person locations (θ). Conversely, if we assume that the person parameters are known, then Equation 4 can be solved iteratively to obtain maximum likelihood estimates of the item locations (δ). Baker and Kim (2004) provide detailed examples of how MLE estimates are obtained. The method is called joint maximum likelihood because of the stepwise process that involves the "joint" or simultaneous estimation of both person and item location on the latent variable.

In practice, the log of Equation 4 is maximized in order to obtain item or person locations. The log likelihood equation is

$$L = \sum_{i=1}^{L} X_i \ln(P_i) + (1 - X_i)^{1-x_i} \ln(1 - P_i) \qquad [6]$$

In order to maximize this likelihood function for persons, the first and second derivatives of L with respect to person location (θ) are needed. The first derivative is

$$\frac{dL}{d\theta} = \sum_{i=1}^{L}(X_i - P_i) \tag{7}$$

while the second derivative is

$$\frac{d^2L}{d\theta^2} = -\sum_{i=1}^{L}P_i(1 - P_i). \tag{8}$$

Newton-Raphson iterations can be used to obtain the maximum likelihood estimate of q as follows:

$$\theta^{k+1} = \theta^k - \frac{\sum_{i=1}^{L}(X_i - P_i^k)}{-\sum_{i=1}^{L}P_i^k(1 - P_i^k)} \tag{9}$$

where θ^k is an initial estimate of the person's location, and θ^{k+1} is the updated estimate. The k–iterations can be continued until the changes between the θs reach a suitably small value, such as .001. The steps for the JMLE Method are summarized in Tables 7.11 and 7.12.

Table 7.11 Steps in the Preliminary Estimation of Person and Item Locations with Joint Maximum Likelihood Estimation Method

Step	Equations	Description
Preliminary Item Logits		
I1	$p_j = \sum_{i=1}^{N} x_{ij} / N$	Mean of item-correct scores [$p_j \equiv$ p-value for item j]
I2	$\hat{\delta}_j = \ln[(1 - p_j)/p_j]$	Preliminary estimates of item logits
I3	$\overline{\delta} = \sum_{j=1}^{L} \hat{\delta}_j / L$	Mean of item logits
I4	$\hat{\delta}_{j[0]} = \ln[(1 - p_j)/p_j] - \overline{\delta}$	Centered estimates of item logits iteration=[0]
Preliminary Person Logits		
P5	$p_i = \sum_{j=1}^{L} x_{ij} / L$	Mean of person-correct scores [$p_i \equiv$ percent-correct score for person i]
P6	$\hat{\theta}_{i[0]} = \ln[p_i/(1 - p_i)]$	Preliminary estimates of person logits iteration = [0]

Note. The PROX estimates of person locations and item difficulties can also be used as starting values for the iterative process.

Table 7.12 Newton-Raphson Iterations to Adjust Item Difficulties (Steps I1 to I6) and Person Measures (P1 to P5): Joint Maximum Likelihood Estimation Method

Step	Equations	Description
Iterations to adjust item locations (I1 to I5)		
I1	$s_j = \sum_{i=1}^{N} x_{ij}$	Item-correct scores [s_j is the number correct score for item j and N is the number of persons]
I2	$p_{ij[k]} = \dfrac{\exp(\hat{\theta}_i - \hat{\delta}_{j[k]})}{1 + \exp(\hat{\theta}_i - \hat{\delta}_{j[k]})}$	Expected p_{ij} at iteration = [k]
I3	$A_{j[k]} = \dfrac{\sum_{i=1}^{N-1} p_{ij[k]} - s_j}{-\sum_{i=1}^{N-1} p_{ij[k]}(1 - p_{ij[k]})}$	Adjustment to item difficulties at step [k]
I4	$\hat{\delta}_{j[k+1]} = \hat{\delta}_{j[k]} - A_{j[k]}$	Adjusted estimates of item difficulties at iteration [k+1]
I5	$\left|\hat{\delta}_{j[k+1]} - \hat{\delta}_{j[k]}\right| < .01$	Repeat steps I2, I3 and I4 until absolute value of differences between item difficulties is small
I6	$\hat{\delta}_{j[k]} - \overline{\delta}_{[k]}$	Re-center item difficulties
Iterations to adjust person measures (P1 to P5)		
P1	$r_i = \sum_{j=1}^{L} x_{ij}$	Person-correct scores [r_i is raw score person i and L is the number of items]
P2	$p_{ij[k]} = \dfrac{\exp(\hat{\theta}_{i[k]} - \hat{\delta}_j)}{1 + \exp(\hat{\theta}_{i[k]} - \hat{\delta}_j)}$	Expected p_{ij} at iteration = [k]
P3	$A_{i[k]} = \dfrac{r_i - \sum_{i=1}^{L-1} p_{ij[k]}}{-\sum_{i=1}^{L-1} p_{ij[k]}(1 - p_{ij[k]})}$	Adjustment to person locations at iteration [k]
P4	$\hat{\theta}_{i[k+1]} = \hat{\theta}_{i[k]} - A_{i[k]}$	Adjusted estimates of person location at iteration [k+1]
P5	$\left|\hat{\theta}_{i[k+1]} - \hat{\theta}_{i[k]}\right| < .001$	Repeat steps P2, P3 and P4 until absolute value of differences between person locations is small

Repeat steps I1–I6 and P1–P5 until estimates converge

2. MML Method

The use of Marginal Maximum Likelihood (MML) Methods for estimating the parameters of general item response models was proposed by Bock and Aiken (1981). It is also called the EM algorithm because the procedure includes two steps: estimation and maximization. Thissen (1982) describes how the MML Method can be used to estimate item parameters of the dichotomous Rasch model.

One of the distinctive features of the MML Method is that the prior distribution of person measures is assumed to be known in advance. This is similar to the use of the assumption of a normal distribution with the PROX Method described earlier. There are also versions of the MML Method that provide an iterative structure that allows the updating of the prior distribution of person measures based on the empirical distribution of person measures in the observed data set.

The MML Method is currently used as the estimation method in the Con-Quest computer program developed by Wu, Adams, and Wilson (1997). The MML Method is the most commonly used estimation method with 2PL and 3PL models as implemented by computer programs such as BILOG and PARSCALE (du Toit, 2003). It is also possible with these software packages to estimate the parameters of Rasch models. The user should be cautious when working with and interpreting the parameters from computer programs that were not specifically developed based on the underlying principles of Rasch models and the requirements of invariant measurement. For example, some of the computer programs do not set the slope parameter to 1.00, but instead estimate an average slope parameter that is held constant across items to mimic a Rasch model. Another area of caution when using non-Rasch dedicated software is that the anchoring of the estimates is based on setting the mean of the person distribution to zero, rather than the convention used in Rasch software to set the mean of the item difficulties to zero.

3. CML Method

Rasch (1960/1980) suggested another method for estimating person and item locations that takes full advantage of the separation property of Rasch models. The Conditional Maximum Likelihood (CML) Method for estimation of the parameters in the Rasch model takes full advantage of the unique properties of this class of measurement models. The CML Method is the best theoretically, but it has been found to be relatively inefficient computationally. The basic issue is that round-off errors tend to accumulate in calculating some of the elementary symmetric functions that are required for fully conditioning out the parameters. CML Method is not suitable for estimating parameters in the 2PL or 3PL measurement models.

Recent advance in numerical methods have addressed many of the computational challenges (Linacre, 2004a; Verhelst & Glas, 1995). This method of estimation has also been called the Fully Conditional (FCON) Method by Wright and his colleagues (Wright, 1980). Anderson (1973) provides a description of the CML Method, and Andrich (1988) uses a small example to illustrate in detail how to calculate CML estimates for the dichotomous Rasch model.

4. Person Measurement: Illustrative Data Analysis of MLE Method (Iterative Method)

This section illustrates the use of a maximum likelihood method for estimating the person parameters of the Dichotomous Model. In order to provide sufficient detail regarding the estimation method, the focus in this illustration is on person measurement with the item locations defined as known in advance. The reader should also recall that item calibration and person measurement usually have different amounts of data to use in the estimation process. In other words, the item locations are usually estimated with more precision as compared to the person locations.

It is important to consider the distinction between probability and likelihood as concepts in statistics. Probability requires no data and essentially provides an ideal perspective or prediction regarding possible future events. Likelihood is tied to real and observed data with the underlying question: what is the probability in this particular case with this specific measurement model of observing these empirical data? In other words, what is the likelihood of observing these real data given the statistical model? Theoretical statements and predictions are probabilities, while observed data leads to statements regarding the likelihood of the observed data given a particular theory or statistical model.

There are a variety of maximum likelihood estimation (MLE) methods that can be adapted for estimating the location of a person on the line when the calibrations of the item difficulties are fixed and viewed as known values. One of the most popular methods is the Joint Maximum Likelihood Estimation (JMLE) Method. This section illustrates the person estimation part of the "joint" MLE method. Other methods used to estimate person locations include modal a posteriori (MAP; Bock & Aiken, 1981), marginal maximum likelihood (MML; Bock & Aiken, 1981), expected a posteriori (EAP; Bock & Aiken, 1981), and weighted likelihood (WL; Warm, 1989) estimators. Plausible values are frequently used in large-scales assessment as a way to highlight uncertainty in the estimates of person locations on the latent variable (Adams & Wu, 2002). There have been several robust methods proposed for estimating person location parameters, such as a biweight estimator (Mislevy & Bock, 1982) and a robust jackknife estimator (Wainer & Wright, 1980).

In this section, items are viewed as being pre-calibrated with known item locations (item difficulties). Four items are used in this section to illustrate the MLE Method. As pointed out earlier, the raw score (sum of correct or positive responses for the dichotomous items) is a sufficient statistic. There are 16 possible response patterns possible with four items that yield five possible raw scores. The possible response patterns are shown below:

Raw score	Item Response Pattern
4	[1111]
3	[1110] [1101] [1011] [0111]
2	[1100] [1010] [0110] [1001] [0101] [0011]
1	[1000] [0100] [0010] [0001]
0	[0000]

The item response functions for each item can be used to obtain a likelihood function. Since the Rasch model requires local independence given each person location, the probabilities of a correct or positive response can be multiplied to obtain the likelihood function. For the Dichotomous Model, the probability of observing a response pattern (P) is

$$P = \prod_{i=1}^{L} P_i^{x_i} (1 - P_i)^{1-x_i} \qquad [10]$$

where x_i represents the dichotomous response of each person to item i with $x = 1$ for a correct or positive response and $x = 0$ for an incorrect or negative response, P_i is the probability of a correct response ($x = 1$) based on the Rasch model, and L is the number of items. Since the item parameters are defined as known in this section, the likelihood of observing a particular response pattern can be obtained from Equation 10. This is shown in the Table 7.13.

The first column gives the four item locations (item difficulties), the second column is the observed response pattern [1110], while the next column provides a graphical representation of the item response functions.

There are four ways to obtain a raw score of three. Within the context of the Dichotomous Model, the most likely response pattern for a score of 3 is [1110] on these four items. The likelihood functions are presented in Table 7.14.

There are several things to note. First of all, [1110] has the highest likelihood based on the given item locations. Next, the same score of 3 maps to the same location on the scale of 1.39 logits regardless of score pattern. Finally, it is important to note that the mode of the likelihood function defines the "best" estimate of person location from the perspective of maximum likelihood estimation, and that this mode is the same regardless of response patterns for all summed scores of "3." Similar displays can be constructed for other scores and responses patterns. For each score group, the Guttman patterns [1000], [1100], and [1110] have the highest likelihoods.

Table 7.13 Item response functions for four items and score of three

Item locations	Responses (x=0,1)	Item response functions
1.50	0	
.50	1	
-.50	1	
-1.50	1	

Score=3

Likelihood Function

Table 7.14   Likelihood Functions for Various Responses Patterns for Scores that Sum to Three

Response Patterns (Score = 3)	Likelihood Functions
[1110]	Likelihood Function
[1101]	Likelihood Function
[1011]	Likelihood Function
[0111]	Likelihood Function

Graphical displays provide a useful way to visualize the likelihood function, and they can be used to estimate the mode of the likelihood function. However, numerical methods provide the necessary machinery to actually calculate the mode of this function that defines the person location on the latent variable. The most common numerical method is called the Newton-Raphson algorithm. This is an iterative procedure that finds the maximum value of the curve that represents the likelihood function in the graphical displays. These iterative steps are shown in Table 7.15.

Table 7.15 Newton-Raphson Iterations to Obtain Maximum Likelihood Estimate of Person Location

Item locations	Response Patterns	Probability of a Correct Response	Probability of an Incorrect Response	Information	Residual
First iteration					
Items	x	p	1-p	p(1-p)	x-p
1.50	0.00				
0.50	1.00				
-0.50	1.00				
-1.50	1.00				
Theta=	0.00		Sum	A	B
Adj(θ)=B/A					
Second iteration					
Items	x	p	1-p	p(1-p)	x-p
1.50	0.00	0.18	0.82	0.15	-0.18
0.50	1.00	0.38	0.62	0.24	0.62
-0.50	1.00	0.62	0.38	0.24	0.38
-1.50	1.00	0.82	0.18	0.15	0.18
Theta=	1.30			0.77	1.00
Adj(θ)=B/A	1.30				
Third Iteration					
Items	x	p	1-p	p(1-p)	x-p
1.50	0.00	0.45	0.55	0.25	-0.45
0.50	1.00	0.69	0.31	0.21	0.31
-0.50	1.00	0.86	0.14	0.12	0.14
-1.50	1.00	0.94	0.06	0.05	0.06
Theta=	1.39			0.64	0.06
Adj(θ)=B/A	0.09				

(*continued*)

Table 7.15 Continued

Item locations	Response Patterns	Probability of a Correct Response	Probability of an Incorrect Response	Information	Residual
Fourth iteration					
Items	x	p	1-p	p(1-p)	x-p
1.50	0.00	0.47	0.53	0.25	-0.47
0.50	1.00	0.71	0.29	0.21	0.29
-0.50	1.00	0.87	0.13	0.11	0.13
-1.50	1.00	0.95	0.05	0.05	0.05
Theta=	1.39			0.62	0.00
Adj(θ)=B/A	0.00				

In order to illustrate the Newton-Raphson iterations, the example with four items is continued. Table 7.15 presents the details of for obtaining the ML estimates for a person with a score of 3 with a response pattern of [1110]. Column 1 gives the item locations, while column 3 gives the response pattern. Columns 3 to 6 show the results for the probabilities of correct and incorrect responses, item information and residuals in that order. An estimate of the standard error for the person location is given by the inverse of the square root of the information:

$SE(\theta) = 1 / \sqrt{\text{Information}}$.

Discussion and Summary

The difference between a parameter and an estimate of it must, however, be kept in mind. A parameter is a quantity entering into the description of a probability model.

(Rasch, 1960/1980, p. 77)

Rasch reminds us of the distinction between parameters and estimates. Chapter 3 focused on the ideal-type view of measurement models that can meet the requirements of invariant measurement. The values in these ideal-type models for measurement are parameters. This chapter focused on the estimation of parameters in Rasch models from observed data. This chapter provides an overview of several estimation methods used within the context of Rasch measurement theory using the Dichotomous Model. Issues related to various estimation methods were described and various methods of numerical analyses briefly presented for the statistical estimation of the parameters of Rasch models. Estimation for measurement models reflects the statistical problem of obtaining parameter estimates based on observed data. Table 7.16 provides a

Table 7.16 Summary of estimation methods for Rasch measurement models

Estimation Method	Distinctive Features	Primary Focus/ Notes	Key References
LOG Method	Non-iterative	Historical interest	Rasch (1960/1980)
PROX Method	Non-iterative	Item calibration Person measurement	Cohen (1979)
PAIR Method	Non-iterative	Item calibration	Choppin (1968) Garner & Engelhard (2000)
CML Method	Iterative	Item calibration	Rasch (1960/1980) Anderson (1973)
MML Method	Iterative	Item calibration	Bock & Aiken (1981) Thissen (1982)
JMLE	Iterative	Item calibration Person measurement	Wright & Panchapakesan (1969)
Biweight estimates	Iterative	Person measurement (robust estimator)	Bock & Mislevy (1982)
Jackknife estimates	Iterative	Person measurement (robust estimator)	Wainer & Wright (1980)
EAP estimates	Iterative	Person measurement (mean of likelihood function)	Bock & Aiken (1981)
MAP estimates	Iterative	Person measurement (median of likelihood function)	Bock & Aiken (1981)
Plausible value estimates	Iterative	Person measurement (Large-scale international tests)	Adams & Wu (2002)
Warm estimates	Iterative	Person measurement (unbiased estimator)	Warm (1989)

summary of the estimation methods that have been used with Rasch measurement models.

One of the main points of this chapter is that various estimation methods tend to yield invariant locations of item and person parameters. Point estimates tend to be comparable for most data sets that are well-behaved, while the estimation of uncertainty based on standard errors of the estimates can vary significantly depending on sample-size and underlying assumptions that vary across the numerical methods used to obtain parameter estimates. It is also important to remember that estimates of model parameters and model-data fit are inherently dependent on the data set being analyzed. In this situation, we are drawing inferences about whether aspects of an ideal-type model (Rasch measurement model in this case) yield invariant measurement within the context of a particular data set. Rasch (1977) used the phrase "specific objectivity" to remind researchers of the sample-dependent aspects of estimates and model-data fit within the context of a particular observed data set In theory, Rasch models work perfectly, while invariant measurement remains a hypothesis to be evaluated regarding how well Rasch models function in a particular situation.

The estimation methods described in this chapter were selected because they illustrate key features of the Rasch model. Baker and Kim (2004) provide clear descriptions of other estimation methods with illustrative computer programs written in BASIC. Some of the other methods of estimation that have been proposed are: Log-linear Method (Kelderman, 1984) and Minimum Logit Chi-square Method (Linacre, 2004a).

A key question that remains to be addressed is: How well does the Rasch model work for a particular observed data set? There are several aspects to this question: How precise and accurate are the estimated parameters of the model? Is the model-data fit (quality control) adequate to meet the requirements of invariant measurement? How "good" is "good enough" to make the judgment that invariant measurement has be realized for the observed data set? The discussion of how to answer these questions is the focus of the next chapter.

Chapter 8

Model-Data Fit for the Dichotomous Rasch Models

Models should not be true, but it is important that they are applicable.
(Rasch, 1960/1980, pp. 37–38)

Model-data fit within the framework of the dichotomous Rasch model is the focus of this chapter. Once estimates are obtained for the parameters of the Rasch model using an estimation method from Chapter 7, then the next step is to explore model-data fit in order to evaluate whether or not the requirements of invariant measurement have been approximated within a particular data set. As pointed out in Chapter 3, Rasch models represent an ideal-type view of measurement theory that meets perfectly the requirements of invariant measurement. In practice, the researcher obtains estimates of the parameters for a particular Rasch model as shown in Chapter 7. These parameter estimates represent the locations of items and persons on a variable map. Once a set of parameter estimates is available, the next step is to examine and evaluate model-data fit. The desirable properties of invariant measurement are only obtained when good model-data fit is achieved. According to Wright (1980),

> Estimation is only half the measurement story, in a sense, the second half. Before we can take estimates or the standard errors seriously, we must verify that the data from which they came are not too unruly to be governed by a measurement model, that they are suitable for measurement. If the data cannot be brought into an order which fits with a measurement models, then we will not be able to use these data for measurement, no matter what we do to them. The requirements for results that we are willing to call measures are specified in the model, and if the data cannot be managed by the model, then the data cannot be used to calibrate items or measure persons. (p. 193)

Wright's comment that data must be "suitable for measurement" has been a bit controversial in the measurement community. It highlights the idea that some data sets may not meet the measurement standards needed to provide useful scales. In some applications, the researcher may want to edit the data to eliminate unusual responses or outliers, and this has been controversial in the measurement community as compared to being a commonly recommended practice in applied statistical analyses. For the perspective of invariant measurement, it is important to recognize and examine residuals and other unexpected values—they do not necessarily have to explicitly included in the measurement model, but it is also not satisfying to eliminate them without consideration of why they are misfitting. As Andrich (1989) has pointed out, it is important to view the process of model-data fit within the context of measurement as addressing the question of whether or not the data are in accord with the requirements of a particular measurement model. Smith (2004) provides a useful overview of fit analyses within the context of Rasch measurement models.

This chapter describes a combination of statistical indices and graphical displays of model-data fit. Ultimately, the researcher in the social, behavioral, and health sciences makes a judgment regarding whether or not the degree of model-data fit is acceptable within the context of the proposed uses, and the interpretative structure that originally motivated the development of the scales. Information obtained from model-data fit analyses provides evidence for the decision regarding whether or not our parameter estimates are "good enough" for the intended uses of the scale. Within the context of this book, the evaluation of *how good is good enough* depends on how well the requirements of invariant measurement are approximated within a particular data set. Theoretically, the Rasch model meets the requirements of invariant measurement perfectly, while the hypotheses related to invariant measurement must be examined within the context of an actual scale being used as a measure with a real data set.

This chapter includes the following sections:

* Brief history of model-data fit for categorical data (overall fit)
* Conceptual framework for model-data fit based on residual analyses
  1. Guttman's Perspective on Model-Data Fit
  2. Model-data fit statistics for dichotomous Rasch Model
* Additional issues related to model-data fit
* Discussion and Summary

Brief History of Model-data Fit for Categorical Data

This section starts with a short general history of model-data fit. This brief history includes an examination of standard indices of fit for categorical data based on Pearson, likelihood ratio chi-squared, and Cressie-Read statistics. Illustrative data analyses exploring the overall fit of the Rasch model are provided for four items from Stouffer and Toby (1951).

In the early 20th century, Pearson (1900) introduced the chi-squared test for examining goodnessof-fit for categorical data (Plackett, 1983). Categorical data can be defined in terms of counts or frequencies that are distributed over cells in a one-way or multi-way contingency table. Pearson (1900) proposed the chi-squared statistic as an approach for testing the fit between a set of expected frequencies and experimentally observed data. Fisher (1924) provided an updated perspective on the Pearson χ^2 statistic, and comprehensive histories of the developments of the statistic are provided by Cochran (1952) and Lancaster (1969).

One of the persistent problems in statistics is the determination of the goodness-of-fit between observed and expected values. The problem is particularly tricky with discrete multivariate data that form the basis for measurement in the social, behavioral, and health sciences. Early work in statistics led to Pearson's chi-square statistic (Pearson, 1900). The chi-square statistic has been quite robust and useful in a variety of applications. Several researchers have proposed adaptations and improvements of chi-square statistics that have ranged from adjustments in the degrees of freedom (Fisher, 1924) to the development of the closely related log likelihood ratio statistic (Wilks, 1935). Unfortunately, the assumptions of the Pearson chi-squared statistic are not always met, and therefore the χ^2 sampling distribution is not necessarily a useful guide for judgments regarding model-data fit.

Read and Cressie (1988) described an approach to goodness-of-fit statistics based on the Power-Divergence (PD) Statistics. These PD statistics can be used to define a family of goodness-of-fit statistics that match earlier fit statistics, such as Pearson's chi-squared statistic. This is a useful way to view goodness-of-statistics because it highlights the common aspects of each of the chi-squared statistics. Engelhard (2008) suggested using this PD statistics, τ^2, with Rasch measurement models based on Cressie and Read (1988). The general form of the PD fit statistics is as follows:

$$\tau^2 = \frac{2}{\lambda(\lambda+1)} \sum_{i=1}^{k} O_i \left[\left(\frac{O_i}{E_i} \right)^{\lambda} - 1 \right] \qquad [1]$$

where O_i is the observed frequency in a cell i, E_i is the expected frequency for cell i based on the model, and k is the number of cells. Goodness-of-fit statistics can be obtained by inserting appropriate λ values in Equation 1. For example, setting λ to 1.00 yields the familiar Pearson X^2, while setting λ close to zero ($\lambda \rightarrow .001$) yields the likelihood ratio G^2 statistic. Setting the λ to .67 yields the Cressie-Read statistic.

We can use Equation 1 to obtain an estimate of the Pearson χ^2 value by setting λ to 1:

$$\chi^2 = \frac{2}{1(1+1)} \sum_{i=1}^{k} O_i \left[\left(\frac{O_i}{E_i} \right)^{1} - 1 \right]$$

The likelihood ratio G^2 can be obtained by setting the lambda value to .001 in Equation 1.

$$G^2 = \frac{2}{.001(.001+1)} \sum_{i=1}^{k} O_i \left[\left(\frac{O_i}{E_i} \right)^{.001} - 1 \right]$$

Finally, the Cressie-Read statistic (1988) can be obtained by setting the lambda value to .67 in Equation 1:

$$CR^2 = \frac{2}{(.67)(1+.67)} \sum_{i=1}^{k} O_i \left[\left(\frac{O_i}{E_i} \right)^{.67} - 1 \right]$$

In order to illustrate the use of these model-data fit values, Table 8.1 shows the frequency data for four items from Stouffer and Toby (1951). Column 1 includes the person scores for the four items including the person location for

Table 8.1

Person Scores (θ)	Item Patterns (4 items)	Observed Freq.	Rasch Probability for Response Patterns	Rasch Expected Freq.
	ABCD			
4	1111	20	---	---
3 (1.52)	1110	38	.830	45.65
	1101	9	.082	4.51
	1011	6	.075	4.12
	0111	2	.013	0.72
2 (-.06)	1100	24	.461	29.04
	1010	25	.408	25.70
	0110	7	.078	4.91
	1001	4	.039	2.46
	0101	2	.007	0.44
	0011	1	.007	0.44
1 (-1.54)	1000	23	.734	26.42
	0100	6	.136	4.90
	0010	6	.120	4.32
	0001	1	.010	0.36
0	0000	42	---	---
		N = 216 N* = 154		Adjusted N* = 154

Adapted from Stouffer, S.A. & Toby, J. 1951. Role conflict and personality. The American Journal of Sociology, 56, 395-406.
Note. Rasch item difficulties are -1.89, -.20, -.10, and 2.20 logits for items A to D respectively. N* represents the number of persons excluding the perfect scores of 0 [0000], and 4 [1111].

scores one, two and three. The next column gives all of the possible patterns for the four items (A, B, C, and D). The third column includes the observed frequency of responses for the 216 persons who responded to these items. Next, the Rasch probability of each response pattern is shown. The fifth column gives the expected frequencies based on the Rasch probabilities for each response pattern. The observed frequencies for each response pattern for Items A, B, C, and D can be compared to the expected frequencies based on the Rasch model. The table below summarizes the obtained estimates for each of the statistics:

Statistic	λ value	Estimate of τ^2	Authors
Chi-squared (χ^2)	1.00	20.37	Pearson (1900)
Likelihood ratio (G^2)	.001	15.16	Wilks (1935)
Cressie-Read (CR^2)	.67	18.23	Cressie & Read (1988)

The 95th percentile of the chi-squared distribution with 13 degrees of freedom is χ^2 (13, p = .05) = 22.36. The value for degrees of freedom is based on the number of cells minus 1. Based on this critical value, we can conclude that the goodness-of-fit is quite good between the observed and expected frequencies based on the Rasch model. The Rasch model provides acceptable model-data fit for the Stouffer and Toby data. These values support the inference that the Rasch model provides good overall or total model-data fit for these data.

The interested reader should consult Read and Cressie (1988) for more information on goodness-of-fit statistics for discrete multivariate data. Agresti (1990) provides a helpful and general overview of categorical data analysis.

Conceptual Framework for Model-Data Fit Based on Residual Analyses

In addition to looking at model-data fit in terms of grouped or frequency data, the Rasch model can also be used to examine the fit of individual person responses to each of the items. This conceptual framework is shown in Figure 8.1. The framework consists of four components. The first component is the observed data (X_{ij} = 0, 1)—dichotomous for this example. Next, a statistical model is fit to the data with the expected values (.00 > P_{ij} > 1.00) based on a particular measurement model and theory regarding the latent variable being constructed. A set of residuals (−1.00 > R_{ij} < 1.00) is obtained next based on the differences between the observed and expected values. This simple framework leads to the research question of "How closely do the observed values match the expected values based on the model?" The next section illustrates this residual-based approach to model-data fit using Guttman scaling (a deterministic ideal-type model), and then the dichotomous Rasch model (a probabilistic ideal-type model).

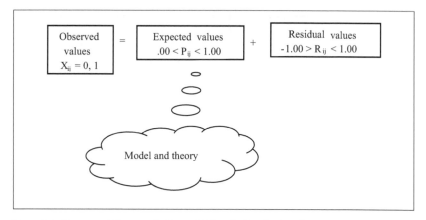

Figure 8.1   *Conceptual framework for model-data fit: Residual analyses.*

I. Guttman's Perspective on Model-Data Fit

Guttman offered a useful general perspective on model-data fit using his deterministic scaling model based on Figure 8.1. Guttman considered the comparative analysis of observed response patterns with the ideal or expected responses as a method for identifying individuals or groups for further study. According to Guttman, "As a matter of fact, a study of the deviants is an interesting by-product of the scale analysis. Scale analysis actually picks out individuals for case studies" (1944, p. 149). These "deviants" define unexpected cases that may yield important new understandings of both items and persons. The study of deviants and apparently anomalous results can play an important role in scientific progress (Kuhn, 1970). Guttman's view of "deviants" as candidates for case studies provides an essential bridge between quantitative and qualitative analyses that can be used to define a mixed-methods approach to disciplined inquiry for the social, behavioral, and health sciences.

There are a variety of methods that have been proposed for examining model-data fit for Guttman scales. Discussions of these model-data fit indices for evaluating Guttman scales are provided by Cliff (1983) and Mokken (1971). The methods proposed for evaluating Guttman scales involve comparisons between observed and expected or perfect response patterns. Guttman (1950) originally proposed a coefficient of reproducibility as follows:

> The amount by which a scale deviates from the ideal scale patterns is measured by a *coefficient of reproducibility* [italics in the original] … It is secured by counting up the number of responses which would have been predicted wrongly for each person on the basis of his scale score, dividing these errors by the total number of responses and subtracting the results fraction from 1 … An acceptable approximation to a perfect scale has been arbitrarily set at 90 per cent reproducibility. (p. 77)

Guttman's coefficient of reproducibility (GCR) is defined as:

GCR = 1 − (total number of errors/total number of responses)   [2]

  = 1 − (E/NL)

where E represents an error count, N is the number of persons and L is the number of items. This definition of reproducibility follows a similar definition by Goodenough (1944), and often is called the Guttman-Goodenough coefficient of reproducibility (Mokken, 1971).

The calculation of the GCR index can be illustrated with the Stouffer and Toby (1951) data set. Table 8.2 provides another way to view the Stouffer and Toby (1951) data set using the conceptual framework in Figure 8.1. The first three columns provide the person scores, item patterns and the observed frequencies for each item response pattern. The next twelve columns provide the observed responses (columns 4–7), expected responses based on the Guttman pattern for each person score (columns 8–11), and residuals obtained by subtracting the expected from observed responses (columns 12–15). The last column in Table 8.2 shows the absolute values for residuals. The sum of these residuals weighted by the observed frequencies is 140. Using Equation 2, the estimate of the GCR index is as follows:

$$1-[140/ (216*4)] = .84$$

This value is lower than Guttman's recommended value of .90, and it suggests that further analyses of residuals may provide additional information to identify unusual cases for further study.

Guttman's approach to model-data fit provides a useful way to conceptualize fit for Rasch measurement models at the individual level of analysis. The residuals obtained by calculating the difference between observed and expected responses derived from the model can also define the most commonly used model-data fit statistics in the Rasch measurement literature. See Engelhard (2005a) for additional details on Guttman scaling, and its connections to Rasch measurement theory.

2. Model-Data Fit Statistics for Dichotomous Rasch Model

This section considers of how various model-data fit indices for categorical data can be adapted, and then used with the dichotomous Rasch Model. Within the context of invariant measurement, data sets that exhibit good fit to the Rasch model yield the desirable characteristics of invariant measurement—item-invariant person measurement and person-invariant item calibration. Specifically, this section reviews the dichotomous Rasch model, and then describes the popular residual-based fit statistics that have been used with this model.

Table 8.2   Guttman Patterns for Four Items

Person Scores	Item Patterns (4 items) ABCD	Freq.	Observed Responses A	B	C	D	Expected Responses A	B	C	D	Guttman Residuals A	B	C	D	Sum of residuals (absolute value)	Weighted sum of residuals
4	1111	20	1	1	1	1	1	1	1	1	0	0	0	0	0	0
3	1110	38	1	1	1	0	1	1	1	0	0	0	0	0	0	0
3	1101	9	1	1	0	1	1	1	1	0	0	0	-1	1	2	18
3	1011	6	1	0	1	1	1	1	1	0	0	-1	0	1	2	12
3	0111	2	0	1	1	1	1	1	1	0	-1	0	0	1	2	4
2	1100	24	1	1	0	0	1	1	0	0	0	0	0	0	0	0
2	1010	25	1	0	1	0	1	1	0	0	0	-1	1	0	2	50
2	0110	7	0	1	1	0	1	1	0	0	-1	0	1	0	2	14
2	1001	4	1	0	0	1	1	1	0	0	0	-1	0	1	2	8
2	0101	2	0	1	0	1	1	1	0	0	-1	0	0	1	2	4
2	0011	1	0	0	1	1	1	1	0	0	-1	-1	1	1	4	4
1	1000	23	1	0	0	0	1	0	0	0	0	0	0	0	0	0
1	0100	6	0	1	0	0	1	0	0	0	-1	1	0	0	2	12
1	0010	6	0	0	1	0	1	0	0	0	-1	0	1	0	2	12
1	0001	1	0	0	0	1	1	0	0	0	-1	0	0	1	2	2
0	0000	42	0	0	0	0	0	0	0	0	0	0	0	0	0	0
		N=216													24	140

Adapted from Stouffer, S.A. & Toby, J. 1951. Role conflict and personality. *The American Journal of Sociology, 56*, 395-406.
Note. Guttman-Goodenough reproducibility coefficient: 1-[140/(216*4)] = .84,

The reader will recall that the operating characteristic (OC) function for the Dichotomous Rasch Model can be written as:

$$\phi_{ni1} = \frac{\exp(\theta_n - \delta_i)}{1 + \exp(\theta_n - \delta_i)} \qquad [3]$$

Equation 3 represents the conditional probability (ϕ_{ni1}) of person n (θ_n) on item i (δ_i) responding with a correct or positive response (x = 1). The differences between person and item locations on the line govern the probability of observing an incorrect/negative response (x = 0) or correct/positive response (x = 1). In essence, the statistical problem is to estimate the row and column values for persons and items that can be used to reproduce the observed responses in a data matrix.

There are several things to remember before describing specific model-data fit methods. First of all, the θ - values and δ - values represent the locations of persons and items on the latent variable (variable map), respectively. It is also important to keep in mind the structure of observed data matrix with dichotomous data (x = 0, 1). The expected values for the cell entries are based on the Dichotomous Model. In other words, estimates of person and item locations can be inserted into the model to obtained expected values for entries in the data matrix. Finally, close fit between observed data and the expected values based on the model is needed to support the inference that invariant measurement has been obtained.

Once estimates for person and item locations are obtained, then Equation 3 can be used to obtain the expected probabilities, P_{ni} , as follows:

$$P_{ni1} = \frac{\exp(\hat{\theta}_n - \hat{\delta}_i)}{1 + \exp(\hat{\theta}_n - \hat{\delta}_i)} \qquad [4]$$

Based on the dichotomous Rasch model in Equation 4, an estimate of the response variances (statistical information), Q_{ni} , can be obtained as follows:

Response variances (statistical information): $\quad Q_{ni} = P_{ni} (1 - P_{ni})$

Score residuals, Y_{ni} , and also standardized residuals, Z_{ni}, can be defined as follows:

Score Residuals: $\qquad Y_{ni} = X_{ni} - P_{ni}$

Standardized Residuals: $\quad Z_{ni} = Y_{ni} / Q_{ni}^{1/2}$

These residuals can be summarized in different ways in order to examine model-data fit for the overall model, as well as for item fit and person fit. Typically, model-data fit is examined using two types of mean square error statistics: Infit and Outfit statistics.

The Outfit statistic is an unweighted mean square statistic that can be calculated separately for persons and items. The Outfit statistic for person n, U_n, is defined as follows:

$$\text{Person Outfit} \qquad U_n = \frac{\sum\limits_{i}^{L} Z_{ni}^2}{L}$$

where L is the number of items. The Outfit statistic for item i, U_i, is defined as:

$$\text{Item Outfit} \qquad U_i = \frac{\sum\limits_{n}^{N} Z_{ni}^2}{N}$$

where N is the number of persons.

The Infit statistics for persons and items can be defined in a similar fashion:

$$\text{Person Infit} \qquad U_i = \frac{\sum\limits_{n}^{N} Z_{ni}^2}{N}$$

$$\text{Item Infit} \qquad V_i = \frac{\sum\limits_{n}^{N} Y_{ni}^2}{\sum\limits_{n}^{N} Q_{ni}}$$

The expected value of these statistic when there is good model-data fit is 1.00 with values less than 1.00 indicating less variation than expected in the modeled responses, and values greater than 1.00 indicating more variation than expected. Infit statistics are information weighted mean square error statistics. The Infit statistics are sensitive to irregular or unexpected responses on the variable map where the item and person locations are well targeted. On the other hand, Outfit statistics are the standard unweighted mean square statistics that are sensitive to unexpected and unusual responses uniformly across the locations of items and persons.

Standardized versions of both Infit and Outfit statistics can also be estimated. The standard errors for Outfit and Infit statistics are as followings:

$$\text{Outfit standard error} \qquad SE_u = \frac{\sum [(1/Q - 4)]^{1/2}}{\sum 1}$$

$$\text{Infit standard error:} \qquad SE_v = \frac{\sum (Q - 4\sum Q^2)^{1/2}}{\sum Q}$$

The standardized mean square statistics can be estimated as follows:

Standardized Outfit $T_u = (U^{1/3} - 1)(3/SE_u) + (SE_u/3)$

Standardized Infit $T_v = (V^{1/3} - 1)(3/SE_v) + (SE_v/3)$

The equations for defining residuals are summarized in Table 8.3, and the equations for the mean square error statistics are summarized in Table 8.4. It is beyond the scope of this text to go into detail regarding the rationale for deriving these standardized mean square error statistics. The reader should consult Wright and Stone (1979) for further details and the justification for interpreting these statistics.

There is debate in the literature regarding the sampling distributions of the standardized model-data fit statistics (Haberman, 2009; Smith, 2004). The mean square based statistics, Infit and Outfit, can be interpreted as effects sizes, while the standardized versions are more likely to be referred to various sampling distributions, such as the chi-square, binomial and t distributions. Much of the debate centers on the issue that the underlying distribution may not be appropriate when the cell sizes being modeled are effectively viewed as cells with small frequencies (N = 1). The underlying philosophy in this book is that all of the statistical indices are essentially continuous indicators of model-data fit that should be interpreted based on "rules of thumb" that develop within a particular context. Graphical displays should also be constructed that highlight additional aspects of model-data fit that may not be easily detected with simple summary statistics. Variable maps, item and person response functions that include observed and expected values, and residual plots should all be combined to develop a deeper understanding of how well invariant measurement has be accomplished with the data set that is the focus of the study being conducted.

Table 8.3   Residuals for Examining Model-Data Fit (Dichotomous Items)

Statistics	*Equations*
Observed Responses	$X_{ni} = 0, 1$
Expected Responses	$P_{ni1} = \dfrac{\exp(\hat{\theta}_n - \hat{\delta}_i)}{1 + \exp(\hat{\theta}_n - \hat{\delta}_i)}$
Response Variances (Information)	$Q_{ni} = P_{ni}(1 - P_{ni})$
Score Residuals	$Y_{ni} = X_{ni} - P_{ni}$
Standardized Residuals	$Z_{ni} = Y_{ni}/Q_{ni}^{1/2}$

Table 8.4   Mean Square Fit Statistics Based on Residuals for Examining Model-Data Fit (Dichotomous Items)

Statistics	*Equations*
Mean Square Outfit Statistics	
Person Outfit	$U_n = \dfrac{\sum\limits_{i}^{L} Z_{ni}^2}{L}$
Item Outfit	$U_i = \dfrac{\sum\limits_{n}^{N} Z_{ni}^2}{N}$
Mean Square Infit Statistics	
Person Infit	$U_i = \dfrac{\sum\limits_{n}^{N} Z_{ni}^2}{N}$
Item Infit	$V_i = \dfrac{\sum\limits_{n}^{N} Y_{ni}^2}{\sum\limits_{n}^{N} Q_{ni}}$
Standard Errors for Outfit and Infit statistics	
Outfit standard error	$SE_u = \dfrac{\sum [(1/Q - 4)]^{1/2}}{\sum 1}$
Infit standard error	$SE_v = \dfrac{\sum (Q - 4\sum Q^2)^{1/2}}{\sum Q}$
Standardized Mean Square Fit Statistics	
Standardized Outfit	$T_u = (U^{1/3} - 1)(3/SE_u) + (SE_u/3)$
Standardized Infit	$T_v = (V^{1/3} - 1)(3/SE_v) + (SE_v/3)$

Note. Outfit is unweighted mean square statistic, while Infit is information weighted mean square error statistic. N is the number of persons and L is the number of items with n used as a person index

In order to illustrate the calculation and use of the Infit and Outfit statistics, we can return to the Stouffer and Toby (1951) data set. Table 8.5 follows the structure of Table 8.2 with Rasch-based expected values and residuals. The expected values are obtained by inserting the estimated item and person location parameters in Equation 4. There are several things to note that are common between Tables 8.2 and 8.5. First of all, the structure of both tables

Table 8.5 Rasch Patterns for Four Items

Person Scores	Item Patterns	Observed Freq.	Observed Responses				Expected Responses				Rasch Residuals			
	ABCD		A	B	C	D	A	B	C	D	A	B	C	D
4	1111	20	1	1	1	1	0.97	0.85	0.84	0.34	0.03	0.15	0.16	0.66
3	1110	38	1	1	1	0	0.97	0.85	0.84	0.34	0.03	0.15	0.16	-0.34
3	1101	9	1	1	0	1	0.97	0.85	0.84	0.34	0.03	0.15	-0.84	0.66
3	1011	6	1	0	1	1	0.97	0.85	0.84	0.34	0.03	-0.85	0.16	0.66
3	0111	2	0	1	1	1	0.97	0.85	0.84	0.34	-0.97	0.15	0.16	0.66
2	1100	24	1	1	0	0	0.86	0.54	0.51	0.09	0.14	0.46	-0.51	-0.09
2	1010	25	1	0	1	0	0.86	0.54	0.51	0.09	0.14	-0.54	0.49	-0.09
2	0110	7	0	1	1	0	0.86	0.54	0.51	0.09	-0.86	0.46	0.49	-0.09
2	1001	4	1	0	0	1	0.86	0.54	0.51	0.09	0.14	-0.54	-0.51	0.91
2	0101	2	0	1	0	1	0.86	0.54	0.51	0.09	-0.86	0.46	-0.51	0.91
2	0011	1	0	0	1	1	0.86	0.54	0.51	0.09	-0.86	-0.54	0.49	0.91
1	1000	23	1	0	0	0	0.59	0.21	0.19	0.02	0.41	-0.21	-0.19	-0.02
1	0100	6	0	1	0	0	0.59	0.21	0.19	0.02	-0.59	0.79	-0.19	-0.02
1	0010	6	0	0	1	0	0.59	0.21	0.19	0.02	-0.59	-0.21	0.81	-0.02
1	0001	1	0	0	0	1	0.59	0.21	0.19	0.02	-0.59	-0.21	-0.19	0.98
0	0000	42	0	0	0	0								

Adapted from Stouffer, S.A. & Toby, J. 1951. Role conflict and personality. *The American Journal of Sociology, 56,* 395-406.

stresses the decomposition of the observed responses into expected and residual values. The expected values for the Guttman scale are based on the classic Guttman pattern, while the expected values for the Rasch scale are based on the dichotomous Rasch model. The residuals in both cases are obtained by subtracting the expected values from the observed values. The major difference relates to methodology used to summarize the residuals.

Table 8.6 provides the response patterns for persons with scores of 3 on the four items from Stouffer and Toby (1951). Columns 1 to 4 provide the scores (all 3s), response patterns that yield a score of 3, person numbers and items (A, B, C and D). Column 5 in Table 8.6 gives the observed responses. Column 6 gives the expected values based on the Rasch model. The reader should note that the expected responses, P_{ij}, are the same over the four items (ABCD): .97, .85, .84, and .34. The Rasch residuals are shown in Column 7. The Rasch variances are shown next, and the standardized Rasch residuals are given in the final column.

There are four response patterns that yield scores of 3. In the observed data, Persons 21, 59, 68 and 74 can be used to illustrate the person fit statistics defined by the Infit and Outfit mean square (MS) statistics. The statistics for these four persons are shown below:

Persons	Patterns ABCD	Scores	Person Location	S.E.	Infit MS	Outfit MS
21	1110	3	1.54	1.39	0.32	0.23
59	1101	3	1.54	1.39	2.25	1.83
68	1011	3	1.54	1.39	2.31	1.97
74	0111	3	1.54	1.39	2.76	8.39

The locations of these four persons are all defined as 1.54 logits (Column 3). The most important thing to note is that the Guttman pattern [1110] reflects the smallest Infit and Outfit MS statistics, while the worst fitting pattern [0111] have larger Infit and Outfit values of 2.76 and 8.39, respectively. Person fit can also be shown graphically with residual plots. Figure 8.2 shows the residual plots for the four response patterns yielding a score of 3.

These standardized residuals can be interpreted as t-statistics with values above 2.00 and below 2.00 suggesting unexpected responses that warrant further study. The last row shows the residual plot for Person 74, and it highlights the unexpected response of this person to Item 1 (Item A).

Similar analyses can also be conducted to summarize item fit. The table below gives the summary statistics for the four items (A, B, C, and D) from Stouffer and Toby (1951).

Table 8.6 Rasch Analyses for Person Scores of 3: Four Items

Scores	Item Patterns ABCD	Persons	Items	Observed Responses	Expected Responses	Rasch Residuals	Rasch Variances (Information)	Standardized Rasch Residuals
3	1110	21	A	1	0.97	0.03	0.03	0.18
		21	B	1	0.85	0.15	0.13	0.42
		21	C	1	0.84	0.16	0.14	0.44
		21	D	0	0.34	-0.34	0.22	-0.71
3	1101	59	A	1	0.97	0.03	0.03	0.18
		59	B	1	0.85	0.15	0.13	0.42
		59	C	0	0.84	-0.84	0.14	-2.27
		59	D	1	0.34	0.66	0.22	1.40
3	1011	68	A	1	0.97	0.03	0.03	0.18
		68	B	0	0.85	-0.85	0.13	-2.39
		68	C	1	0.84	0.16	0.14	0.44
		68	D	1	0.34	0.66	0.22	1.4
3	0111	74	A	0	0.97	-0.97	0.03	-5.59
		74	B	1	0.85	0.15	0.13	0.42
		74	C	1	0.84	0.16	0.14	0.44
		74	D	1	0.34	0.66	0.22	1.40

Adapted from Stouffer, S.A. & Toby, J. 1951. Role conflict and personality. *The American Journal of Sociology, 56*, 395–406.

Response Patterns (Score of 3)	Residual Plots Items (A=1, B=2, C=3, D=4)
1110	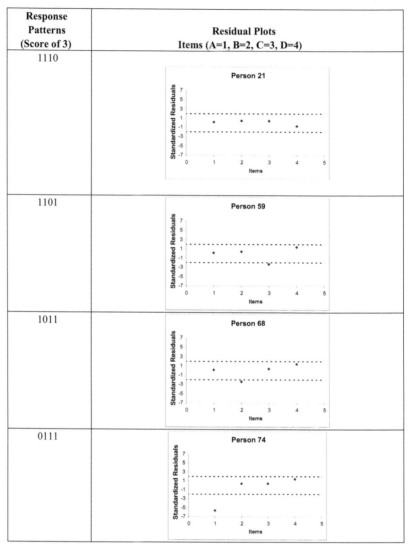
1101	
1011	
0111	

Figure 8.2   Residual plots for Response Patterns (Score of 3).

Items	P-value	Measure	S.E.	Infit MS	Outfit MS
A	0.84	-1.91	0.24	1.05	1.11
B	0.57	-0.21	0.19	0.92	0.89
C	0.55	-0.1	0.19	0.98	0.98
D	0.16	2.21	0.23	1.03	1.11

Since the Infit and Outfit mean square (MS) values are close to the expected value of 1.00, these items represent acceptable fit to the Rasch model. This model-data fit information is shown graphically in Figure 8.3. These item response functions include both the expected values (smooth function lines) from the dichotomous Rasch model, and the observed values within the same figures. These figures are reminiscent of the original displays suggested by Rasch (1960/1980). For example, Figure 6.1 (Panel E) represents acceptable fit according to Rasch with the empirical item response functions not crossing. The Stouffer and Toby (1951) items exhibit acceptable fit with the item response functions not crossing. In addition to the typical Infit and Outfit statistics, it is also possible to create group-based versions of these statistics that

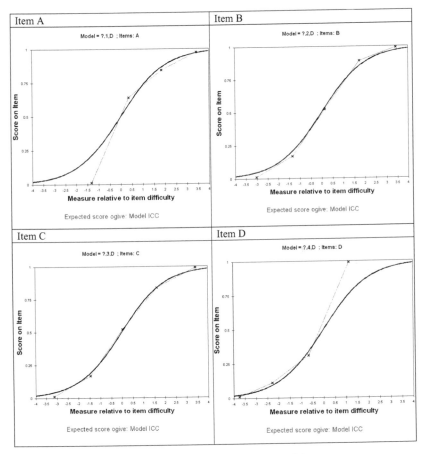

Figure 8.3   Item Response Functions for Items A, B, C, and D.

are directed towards particular hypotheses regarding measurement invariance for person subgroups and item subsets. In each case, the graphical displays can reveal more about model-data fit than simple summary statistics, such as the Infit and Outfit statistics. Engelhard (2008b) provides additional details on conducting these types of analyses.

Additional Issues Related to Model-Data Fit

This chapter has focused on residual-based definitions of model-data fit. There are other issues that should be examined when considering whether or not invariant measurement has been achieved within a particular data set. Swaminathan, Hambleton, and Rogers (2007) and Hambleton and Han (2005) have provided a list of suggested activities to guide practitioners in the assessment of model-data fit. Among their recommendations is that a routine examination of classical indices and statistics (e.g., p-values, item total correlations) be conducted, as well as an examination of model fit using graphical as well as statistical procedures. They also recommend exploring the unidimensionality of the data.

The issue of dimensionality can be conceptualized in a variety of ways. Guttman (1950) suggested that the dimensionality of an observed data set be evaluated based on whether or not a meaningful ordering of persons and items can be obtained—in fact, this was the major motivation for his development of the principles that undergird Guttman scaling. As stated by Guttman (1950), "a simple method for testing a series of qualitative items for unidimensionality" (p. 46) is provided by his reproducibility coefficient. If the items and persons responses exhibit reasonable fit to a Guttman scale, then the ordering of items and persons define a unidimensional scale. This perspective based on response patterns could also provide a logical basis for considering model-data fit to the Rasch model as support for unidimensionality defined from the perspective of invariant measurement.

Another approach for exploratory analyses of dimensionality is to create a scree plot of eigenvalues obtained from the matrix of item inter-correlations. These plots provide a visual display than can be used to guide and inform decisions about whether or not observed data can be approximated by a unidimensional model. Reckase (2009) should be consulted for current perspective on principle component and factor analyses of item data based on multidimensional item response theory. Hattie (1985) summarizes and critiques multiple methods that have been proposed for assessing unidimensionality of test and items.

Figure 8.4 provides a scree plot for the Stouffer and Toby (1951) data. The eigenvalues for these data are 1.775, .866, .713, and .646. The large dip from the first to second eigenvalues supports the inference that data can be adequately represented by a unidimensional model. The first eigenvalue accounts

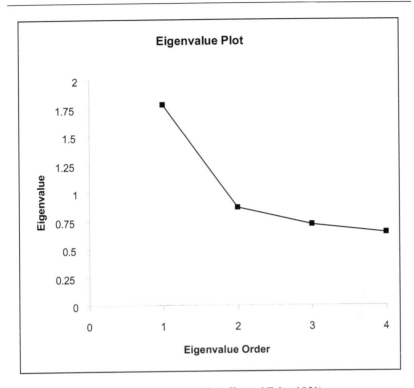

Figure 8.4   Scree Plot of the Four Items (Stouffer and Toby, 1951).

for 44.4% of the variance, and this is above value of 20% of the variance that was suggested as a rule of thumb by Reckase (1979).

It cannot be stressed strongly enough that no single index of model-data fit can detect all of the possible ways that things can go wrong in measurement for the human sciences! It also cannot be stressed enough that how well a particular data set fits a measurement model is based on informed judgments and evaluations of multiple criteria regarding how good is good enough to approximate invariant measurement. Measurement is a process that involves multiple iterations to determine how well our scales and instruments are functioning in a particular context to inform particular decisions.

Discussion and Summary

This chapter explored issues related to model-data fit, and the examination of whether or not the correspondence between the requirements of invariant measurement are judged to be "good enough" to warrant the use of the model with a particular data set. The Rasch model in its ideal-type version meets the requirements of invariant measurement perfectly as designed; however, it is essential to judge whether or not the data set in hand can approximate these requirements. As pointed out by Rasch (1960/1980):

> It may be objected that this model cannot be true. ... that the model is not true is correct, no models are – not even the Newtonian laws. When you construct a model you leave out all the detail which you, with the knowledge at your disposal, consider inessential ... *Models should not be true, but it is important that they are applicable*, and whether they are applicable for any given purpose must of course be investigated. This also means that a model is never accepted finally, only on trial. (pp. 37–38, italics in the original)

As shown in this chapter, the examination of model-data fit can be approached in several different ways. A close fit between observed data and the expected values based on the Rasch measurement model is needed to support the inference that invariant measurement has been obtained. The Rasch measurement community tends to use a residual-based approach as summarized through Infit and Outfit mean square statistics.

Several researchers have criticized the use of these residuals because the estimates of their variances are under-estimated, and this affects the sampling distribution used to interpret the fit statistics (Karabatsos, 2000; Smith & Hedges, 1982). The consequence of this underestimation of the variance is that model agreement may be suggested when agreement is not present. Haberman (2009) has suggested the used of generalized residuals to examine goodness-of-fit for item response models including the dichotomous Rasch model. Future research on model-data fit should explore the use of these generalized residuals. Another promising area for future research is the usefulness of the PD Statistics suggested by Engelhard (2008a). This chapter focused on model-data fit for the dichotomous Rasch model, and these procedures can be generalized for examining model-data fit for other Rasch-measurement models.

Issues related to invariant measurement can also be approached using the theoretical lens of other measurement models. Meredith (1993) and Milsap & Meredith (2007) discuss these issues from the perspective of measurement invariance, while Sijtsma and Molenaar (2002) book should be consulted for how invariant measurement can be examined from the perspective of non-parametric item response theory.

In summary, the key points of this chapter are as follows:

- Interpretations of model-data fit indices require judgments: How good is "good enough"?
- Sampling distributions for fit indices are not exact—rules of thumb and experience-based interpretations are needed for determining substantive significance of results.

- There is no single index of model-data fit that will detect all of the possible disturbances that may affect the measurements encountered in the human sciences.
- Graphical and statistical displays of fit indices offer useful devices for interpreting lack of model-data fit.

Chapter 3 and 10 describe several Rasch measurement models, and methods for estimating the parameters of the dichotomous Rasch model, respectively. Once a Rasch model has been selected and the parameters of the model estimated, then the next step is to analyze how well the observed data match the expected values based on substituting the estimated parameters into the model. Wright and Masters (1982) should be consulted for the extensions of these dichotomous model-data fit indices for the Rating Scale and Partial Credit Models. Linacre (1994) describes the further generalization of model-data fit indices within the context of multifaceted Rasch measurement models. Model-data fit for rater-mediated assessments are addressed in the chapters on rater-mediated assessments.

Part IV

Assessments with Raters

Rater-Invariant Measurement

Chapter 9

Rater-Mediated Assessments

A Conceptual Framework

One of the major trends in assessment in the human sciences is the increased use of constructed-response formats that yield performances that are scored with a rating scale. In educational settings, the use of constructed-response items in combination with selected-response item formats (e.g., multiple-choice items) has become the norm for most assessments. Constructed-response assessments have also been referred to as performance assessments (Lane & Stone, 2006), authentic assessments (Wiggins, 1989), and direct assessments (Huot, 1990). The distinctive feature of constructed-response assessments is that persons are asked to create a performance, such as an essay, that requires a rater to assign a score to the performance that represents the knowledge, skills and achievement level of the person. In order to stress the distinctive features of performance-based assessments, I have used the phrase rater-mediated assessments (Engelhard, 2002). There are a variety of very good reasons for using rater-mediated assessments that include positive influences on teaching and the curriculum of schools; however, insufficient attention has been paid to the potential problems that accrue when rater judgments are introduced into the assessment process.

In early work on performance assessments during the 1980s and 1990s, these assessments were viewed as having little to no measurement problems. The underlying idea was WYSIWYG —what you see is what you get. Multiple-choice and other forms of selected response items were viewed as *indirect* assessments, while performance assessments were viewed as *direct*. The use of ratings from these assessments for variety of high-stakes decisions, such as grade-to-grade promotion and high school graduation soon persuaded researchers (a) that direct assessments, such as written essays and portfolios do have measurement problems, (b) that performance assessments are also "indirect," and (c) that the assignment of ratings that reflect human judgments are mediated through raters. For example, writing competence is a latent variable with the process of locating persons on the latent variable requiring judgment and inferences from raters. It can be argued that performance assessments are even less direct than other forms of assessment because student scores are assigned based on the unique lens that a human judge brings to the measurement process.

The examples and illustrations used in this chapter, as well as Chapters 10 and 11, are primarily based on writing assessment. The application of these general principles generalizes to other rater-mediated assessments. Johnson, Penny, and Gordon (2009) provide a detailed overview of a variety of issues related to performance assessment that includes assessment design, scoring, and validation of tasks and ratings. Lane and Stone (2006) summarize the major topics related to performance assessments in educational settings.

The specific sections of this chapter are:

- Rater-mediated assessments
- Brief comparison of measurement models for raters
- Rater-invariant measurement
  1. Extending the requirements of invariant measurement
  2. Guidelines for evaluating rating category usage
- Many Facet Model
- Using variable maps with rater-mediated assessments
- Summary and discussion

Rater-Mediated Assessments

The conceptual framework that guides my perspective on rater-mediated assessments is broadly based on Brunswik's Lens Model (1952). This model has been used in cognitive psychology to explore human judgment, decision-making and choice activities (Hogarth, 1987). Within the context of writing assessment, the metaphor of a camera including the notion of a "lens" had been used by Carl Brigham (1934) of the College Board:

> The individual reader respects his own judgment and protests against the group judgment. One might almost say that there is a naïve theory of reading which holds that there is an absolute mark and only one mark, which may be affixed to each single effort of each candidate. This theory regards the individual reader as a sort of refined micrometric microscope with exact powers of seeing and gauging, not *a* grade but *the* grade. The opposing theory regards the readers as more or less efficient cameras varying in the efficiency of the lens, focusing devices, and the sensitivity of the film. This year the Board took four pictures of each candidate with this collection of cameras. (p. 30)

Brigham (1934) went further and used this metaphor to guide and evaluate readers who rated the essays: "[The College Board] is now examining its cameras and is about to select the ones which were found most effective" (p. 30). Brunswik (1952) proposed the Lens Model for understanding human perception and judgment. Egon Brunswik was a psychologist who also contributed to the development of the field of ecological psychology with an explicit concern with the role of environments and their interactive influences on human behavior. He coined the term "ecological validity" to stress the contextualized nature and importance of the ecological aspects of human behavior (Brunswik, 1956). Hogarth (1987) adapted Brunswik's Lens Model, and stressed that judgmental accuracy can be interpreted as framing a person's judgment about an event (observed rating) based on a series of cues (domains selected by persons to inform and guide judgments and ratings). Quality and accuracy of the judgments reflect the connections between the observed person judgments and the actual (latent) outcomes. The ecological context includes characteristics of persons (rater characteristics), as well as characteristics of the environment (ecological context). According to Hogarth (1987), a key element for Brunswik was the idea that judgments reflect points of reference that serve as cues to inform decision making. In his words, "most judgments are the result of comparisons with such points of reference or cues" (p. 8). According to Hogarth (1987), Brunswik's Lens Model stresses:

- *Interrelatedness:* judgments are based on an interrelated set of information—judgments are not made in a vacuum;
- *Correspondence:* the relationship between a rater's schema (cognitive map or mental representation of the world) for processing information and reality is an important determinant of judgmental quality;
- *Accuracy:* higher quality judgments are made when there is a close match between a rater's schema and reality;
- *Uncertainty:* all judgments occur within a probabilistic framework;
- *Individual-task interactions*: judgmental accuracy is a function of individual rater characteristics and structure of the task environment.

See Hogarth (1987) for a detailed description of these five key elements. Postman and Tolman (1959) should be consulted for a detailed description of Brunswik's approach to psychology. Hammond and his colleagues are also a good source for learning more about lens models (Hammond, 1996; Hammond & Stewart, 2001).

There are several components of lens models that can illuminate aspects of rater-mediated assessments. First of all, the concept of cues stresses the need for assessment developers to carefully select and monitor aspects of the environment that raters should pay attention to in the rating process. For example, rubrics and other guidelines used for scoring are viewed as cues to the raters. Second, the lens model is grounded in ecological psychology, and it is important to recognize that rater-mediated assessments must be viewed as contextualized within specific assessment environments and systems. And finally, lens models raise issues related to both the precision and accuracy of ratings obtained from a fallible and potentially noisy rating process from human raters.

In order to illustrate how lens models can be used in performance assessment, Panel A in Figure 9.1 is a general representation of the rating process with a prototypical rater-mediated assessment. In this case, the intervening variables (rater characteristic and cues: rubric and rating scale) define the intended lens that guides the definition of the latent variable that is mediated through the intervening variables to yield an observed rating. The rubric can be viewed as a set of descriptors that define the latent variable at various points along the measure or variable map. This figure also indicates that this entire process occurs within a particular ecological context. In essence, the intervening variables define a "lens" that raters use to focus their judgments and inferences about person locations on the latent variable.

Panel B in Figure 9.1 describes a simple lens model for a writing assessment that considers the influences of rater severity (easy to hard) with two

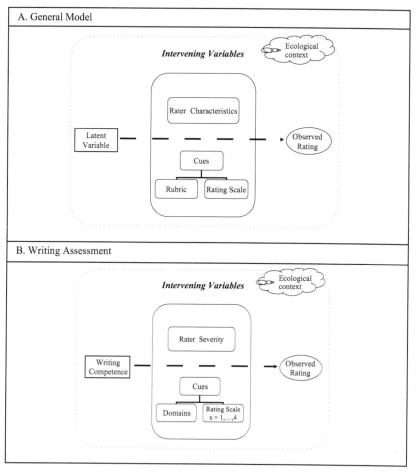

Figure 9.1   Lens Models for Rater-Mediated Assessments.

cues: (a) two writing domains: mechanics and meaning and (b) rating scale with four categories (1 = low to 4 = high). Writing competence is the latent variable, while the purpose of the assessment (high school graduation test in writing) might be an aspect of the ecological context.

Brief Comparison of Measurement Models for Raters

There are a variety of measurement models that have been proposed for examining the quality of ratings and various aspects of rater behaviors. The history of rater-mediated assessments can be viewed in terms of test-score and scaling traditions as described in earlier chapters. Early approaches to modeling ratings include the work of Edgeworth (1890) who described disagreement in scoring English compositions among competent judges. His perspective mirrors the decomposition of observed ratings into true and error components based on classical test theory (test-score tradition). Hoyt (1941) provided another early approach for modeling the rating process from an ANOVA perspective. Wherry (1952) described a systematic theory of ratings that strongly influenced performance appraisal research in applied psychology (Landy & Farr, 1983).

Likert (1932) was an early advocate the use of the test-score tradition for analyzing ratings. Eventually, the test-score tradition for modeling ratings was extended by Generalizability Theory (Cronbach, Gleser, Nanda, & Rajaratnam, 1972). Generalizability Theory continues to be used as a model for examining the generalizability of ratings for performance assessments.

Scaling models for ratings were also being developed during the 20th century. As was pointed out in earlier chapters, much of the measurement research within the scaling tradition had its genesis in the psychophysics of the 19th century. Thurstone (1959) played a major conceptual role by developing his models of judgment and choice (Bock & Jones, 1968). Research on Rasch measurement models for rating scales has been dominated by the research of Andrich (1978) and Masters (1982). Wright and Masters (1982) provide the seminal source for much of the Rasch-based research on rating scale data. Linacre (1994), in his dissertation at The University of Chicago under the direction of Professor Ben Wright, developed a many facet Rasch model that was specifically designed for rater-mediated assessments. This Facets Model underlies the approach to invariant measurement for rater-mediated assessments described in this chapter.

It is beyond the scope of this chapter to provide a complete history of rating scale models. Engelhard (2005) provides a review of item response theory models that have been proposed for rating scale data. Gyagenda and Engelhard (2010) compare the measurement issues encountered in writing assessment when viewed from the perspective of classical test theory (test-score tradition) with the perspective of Rasch measurement theory (scaling tradition). Nonparametric item response theory that represents an extension of Mokken

Scaling to categorical data has been described by Molenaar (1997). Future research is needed to explore the utility of these various models for exploring the psychometric quality of ratings, and their implications for theory and practice within the context of rater-mediated assessments.

Rater-Invariant Measurement

This book has focused on describing invariant measurement and the ways in which invariant measurement can yield measures with desirable measurement properties when the data fits the requirements of an ideal-type model, such as the Rasch model. This section focuses on extending the requirements of invariant measurement to cover issues encountered in rater-mediated assessments, as well as guidelines for examining the psychometric quality of rating scales that are ubiquitous in rater-mediated assessments.

I. Extending the Requirements of Invariant Measurement

This section focuses on the following question: How do the requirements of invariant measurement appear within the context of rater-mediated assessments? To review, the basic five requirements of invariant measurement are:

Person measurement:
1. The measurement of persons must be independent of the particular items that happen to be used for the measuring: Item-invariant measurement of persons.
2. A more able person must always have a better chance of success on an item than a less able person: non-crossing person response functions.

Item calibration:
3. The calibration of the items must be independent of the particular persons used for calibration: Person-invariant calibration of test items.
4. Any person must have a better chance of success on an easy item than on a more difficult item: non-crossing item response functions.

Variable map:
5. Items and person must be simultaneously located on a single underlying latent variable: variable map.

These requirements can be extended to rater-mediated assessments:

Person measurement:
R1. The measurement of persons must be independent of the particular raters that happen to be used for the measuring: Rater-invariant measurement of persons.
R2. A more able person must always have a better chance of obtaining higher ratings from raters than a less able person: non-crossing person response functions.

Rater calibration:
 R3. The calibration of the raters must be independent of the particular persons used for calibration: Person-invariant calibration of raters.
 R4. Any person must have a better chance of obtaining a higher rating from lenient raters than from more severe raters: non-crossing rater response functions.
Variable map:
 R5 Persons and raters must be simultaneously located on a single underlying latent variable: variable map.

These requirements can be extended to cover the domains (items) that are used to define the cues or aspects that guide raters in the assignment of their judgmental ratings. For example, analytic scoring systems typically require raters to rate essays on several domains, such as student proficiency in (a) the mechanics of writing (usage, mechanics and conventions of written language) and (b) the creation of meaningful writing (content, organization and style).

2. Guidelines for Evaluating Functioning of Rating Categories

Assessments in the human sciences include a variety of formats for collecting judgments. One of the most common schemes for collecting these data is in the form of rating scales. The use of rating scales provides a useful format for collecting both self-ratings, as well as judgments collected within the context of rater-mediated assessments. In considering the invariance of rater-mediated assessments, it is important to examine the ways in which the categories are being interpreted and used by the raters. Early work on rating scales viewed the categories indicating fixed locations on the latent variable as shown in Table 9.1. This intended mapping of categories that is assumed when summed ratings are used as scores is shown in Panel A of Table 9.1. Modern researchers have the opportunity to explicitly examine the hypothesis of whether or not the locations of the categories do indeed define equal intervals. Panel B of Table 9.1 illustrates how the categories may actually be used by raters to guide their judgmental processes. In this case, Panel B in Table 9.1 suggests that the assumption of equal intervals would be false. The locations of the thresholds, τ_1, τ_2, and τ_3, (category boundaries) are not equally spaced. Linacre (1999) proposed a set of guidelines for examining the functioning of rating categories. A summary of his seven guidelines are shown in Table 9.2.

 The first guideline is directionality. Directionality addresses the issue of whether or not the rating scale is oriented in the same way as the underlying latent variable. In other words, the category ratings and labels (e.g., 1 = low, 2 = medium, 3 = high) should be aligned with low to high locations on the latent variable. Ultimately, the directionality supports the inference that higher ratings and higher summed ratings indicate higher locations on the latent variable for persons who are assigned the ratings. In addition to defining the categories through the use of rubrics that define an order on the latent variable, empirical

Table 9.1   Implicit and Empirical Rating Categories

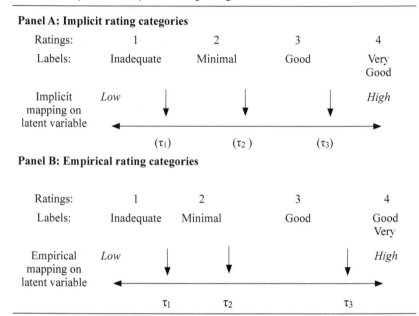

Panel A: Implicit rating categories

Ratings:	1	2	3	4
Labels:	Inadequate	Minimal	Good	Very Good

Implicit mapping on latent variable   *Low*   *High*

(τ_1)   (τ_2)   (τ_3)

Panel B: Empirical rating categories

Ratings:	1	2	3	4
Labels:	Inadequate	Minimal	Good	Good Very

Empirical mapping on latent variable   *Low*   *High*

τ_1 τ_2 τ_3

evidence can be obtained by examining the relationship between the latent variable and the observed and expected scores. The second guideline is that the measures increase monotonically as a function increasing values on the latent variable or measure. Monotonicity can be examined by calculating the average person location that corresponds to each rating category.

Guidelines 3 and 4 address issues related to observed category usage by the raters. Ideally, there should be at least 10 observations or ratings observed in each category (Guideline 3). It is also useful to have a regular distribution of ratings across categories (Guideline 4). For example, a uniform distribution might be desirable for category usage by the raters; however, there are other distributions of ratings across the categories that can yield stable calibrations of the category coefficients. The observed distribution of ratings over categories can be examined to check on Guidelines 3 and 4.

Researchers should also examine model-data fit related to categories (Guideline 5). As pointed out in earlier chapters, model-based approaches based on the Rasch model can be evaluated with mean square statistics that use residual analyses to check model-data fit. Linacre (1999) recommends Outfit mean square statistics of less than 2.00 as an indication of acceptable model-data fit for rating scales.

The next two guidelines deal with the locations of the estimated threshold parameters on the latent variable. Guideline 6 addresses the issue of threshold order. Andrich (1978a, b) has argued for ordered thresholds that reflect the

Table 9.2   Guidelines for Examining Rating Scale Category Usage

Index	Guidelines	Statistical and graphical analyses
1	Directionality: Rating categories aligned with latent variable (construct)	Examine a plot of observed/ expected ratings on latent variable
2	Monotonicity: person locations on latent variable increase with rating categories	Calculate average person location for each category
3	Category usage: 10 or more observations per category	Examine frequency distributions over categories
4	Distribution of ratings: Regular distribution of ratings across categories	Examine frequency distributions over categories
5	Fit of rating scale to Rasch model	Identify Outfit mean square statistics less than 2.00
6	Threshold order: Locations of threshold reflect the intended order of categories	Create a variable map with threshold locations
7	Threshold locations: Locations of thresholds are distinctive	Evaluate threshold differences between locations: $1.40 < \tau_k - \tau_{k-1} < 5.00$ logits

Note. τ is defined as the threshold parameter.

intended order of the categories. Disorder implies lack of scale invariance and affects ordering of persons on the latent variable. Andrich, de Jong, and Sheridan (1997) provide a useful set of substantive and diagnostic recommendations for exploring crossing category response functions. Category response functions represent the relationship between the probabilities associated with each rating category as a function of the latent variable.

In addition to examining threshold order, the usefulness of a rating scale is influenced by how far apart the thresholds are on the latent variable. Guideline 7 suggests that threshold locations should be distinctive. One way to conceptualize a rating scale is as a set of dichotomous items that reflect the probability of moving across adjacent categories. For example, a three-category scale can be viewed as being composed of two dichotomous items that reflect the transition from category 1 to 2, and category 2 to 3. In other words, a three-category rating scale may carry as much information as two multiple-choice items under some conditions. Huynh (1994, 1996) has done extensive work on these conditions, and based on this research Linacre (1999) recommended that differences between threshold parameters, τ_k, should have a value greater than 1.40 and less than 5.00 logits. A useful way to view the effects of category spacing is to examine category information functions. When the thresholds are too close or too far apart, there are distinctive patterns that are visible in the category information functions. Category information response functions are defined in Linacre (1999).

Many Facet Model

A general version of the Many Facet (MF) model that can be used for analyzing rater-mediated assessment can be written as:

$$\phi_{nmik} = \frac{P_{nmik}}{P_{nmik-1} + P_{nmik}} = \frac{\exp(\theta_n - \lambda_m - \delta_i - \tau_k)}{1 + \exp(\theta_n - \lambda_m - \delta_i - \tau_k)} \tag{1}$$

and the category response function as follows:

$$\pi_{nmij} = \frac{\exp\left[\sum_{j=0}^{k}(\theta_n - \lambda_m - \delta_i - \tau_k)\right]}{\sum_{r=0}^{m_i}\exp\left[\sum_{j=0}^{r}(\theta_n - \lambda_m - \delta_i - \tau_k)\right]} \tag{2}$$

This can be presented in log-odds format that highlights the linear structure of the logistic model:

$$Ln\left(\frac{P_{nmik}}{P_{nmik-1}}\right) = \theta_n - \lambda_i - (\delta_i + \tau_k) = \theta_n - \lambda_m - \delta_i - \tau_k \tag{3}$$

where

P_{nmik} = probability of person n being rated k on domain i by rater m,
P_{nmik-1} = probability of person n being rated k–1 on domain i by rater m,
θ_n = judged location of person n,
λ_m = severity of rater m,
δ_i = judged difficulty of domain i, and
τ_k = judged difficulty of rating category k relative to category k–1.

The rating category coefficient, τ_k, is not considered a facet in the model. It represents the threshold value of moving between adjacent rating categories as shown in Table 9.1.

Based on the MF model presented in Equation 3, the probability of person n being rated k on domain i by rater m with a rating category coefficient of τ_k is given as

$$\pi_{nmik} = exp\,[k\,(\theta_n - \lambda_m - \delta_i - \tau_k) - \Sigma\tau_k]\,/\,\gamma \tag{4}$$

where τ_1 is defined to be zero , and g is a normalizing factor based on the sum of the numerators. The normalizing factor is used to assure the probabilities fall between .00 and 1.00. As written in Equation 3, the category coefficients, τ_k, represent a Rating Scale model (Andrich, 1978) with category coefficients fixed across domains. Analyses using the Partial Credit model (Masters, 1982) with the category coefficients allowed to vary across facets can be designated by various subscripts on τ_k. For example, τ_{ik}, would indicate that raters used the categories on the rating scale when assigning ratings for domain i in a different way than they used the categories when assigning ratings for a different domain. In other words, different raters may not share a common understanding of what each category means, and they may be using the categories differently when assigning ratings.

$$P_{nmik} = exp\,[k\,(\theta_n - \lambda_m - \delta_i - \tau_k) - \Sigma\tau_k]\,/\,\gamma \qquad [5]$$

The Facets computer program (Linacre, 2007) can be used to obtain estimates for the parameters in Equation 4, and then the estimates of these parameters can be used in Equation 5 to obtain the expected ratings of P_{nmik}. As was the case for the Dichotomous Model, model-data fit (Chapter 8) can be examined using residuals based on discrepancies between the expected values obtained from the Facets Model and the observed ratings.

The generic Many Facet Model in Equation 3 can be specified to represent several common scoring contexts for rater-mediated assessments. Some illustrative models are shown in Table 9.3. The parameters in the MF model are θ_n (judged writing location of person n, λ_m (severity of rater m), δ_i (judged severity of domain i), and τ_k (judged difficulty of rating category k relative to category k–1). In each of these models, the category coefficients can be parameterized to implement a rating-scale model or partial credit model. This list is meant to be illustrative rather than an exhaustive categorization of all Rasch models for rater-mediated assessments. The Facets Manual (Linacre, 2007) and McNamara (1996) provide numerous illustrations and other Rasch models that may be suitable for different rating procedures.

The MF model is a unidimensional model with a single person parameter (location on the latent variable) that represents the object of measurement, and a collection of other facets, such as raters and domains. As with other Rasch models, if the data fit the model, then it is possible to obtain invariant estimates of person, rater and item locations on the latent variable.

Table 9.3   Scoring Contexts and the Many Facet Model for Rater-Mediated Aassessments

Scoring context	*Many Facet Model*
Multiple raters using one domain (holistic scoring)	$\mathrm{Ln}\,[P_{nmk}\,/\,P_{nmk\text{-}1}] = \theta_n - \lambda_m - \tau_k$
One rater using multiple domains (analytic scoring)	$\mathrm{Ln}\,[P_{nik}\,/\,P_{nik\text{-}1}] = \theta_n - \delta_i - \tau_k$
Multiple raters using multiple domains (analytic scoring)	$\mathrm{Ln}\,[P_{nmik}\,/\,P_{nmik\text{-}1}] = \theta_n - \lambda_m - \delta_i - \tau_k$

Using Variable Maps with Rater-Mediated Assessments

Results from Rasch analyses using the MF Model can be represented graphically in variable maps. One of the goals of invariant measurement is to create a variable map that can serve as an organizing concept for viewing the measures being created by the developer of an assessment. Variable maps provide visual displays of the underlying latent variable with simultaneous location of both domains and persons on a line that represents the construct being measured. Variable maps provide visual displays that answer the following question: What is the latent variable (construct) being measured?

Variable maps are also useful for representing rater-mediated assessments. Figure 9.2 provides a prototypical variable map for rater-mediated assessments. As with all variable maps, Column 1 provides the units for the measuring instrument on a logit scale. Column 2 provides the first step in the

What is the latent variable (construct)?

Logit Scale	Persons	Raters	Domains	Rating Scale Structure
	[High]	*[Severe]*	*[Hard]*	*[High ratings]*
5.00				
4.00	High values on the latent variable			*4=very good*
3.00				
2.00				*3=good*
1.00				
.00	Midrange values on the latent variable	*[Average raters]*	*[Moderately difficult domains]*	
-1.00				*2=minimal*
-2.00				
-3.00				
-4.00	Low values on the latent variable			*1=inadequate*
-5.00				
	[Low]	*[Lenient]*	*[Easy]*	*[Low ratings]*

What is the response format or rating scale used?
  o *Dichotomous (x=0, 1)*
  o *Polytomous (x=0, 1, 2, 3 ...)*

Figure 9.2   Prototypical Variable Map for Rater-Mediated Assessments.

operational definition of our latent variable. The researcher must develop a conception, definition and description of the characteristics of persons who have low, moderate, and high levels on the latent variable. In the case of rater-mediated assessments, these descriptions are embodied in the cues and rubrics used to guide the raters in the assignment of ratings. For example, if the construct is communicative competence in writing, then the researcher begins by defining this latent variable in terms of a vision of what students need to know and be able to do at different levels on the latent variable. This vision is used to select representative essays or papers that correspond to locations on the construct. These defining essays can serve as benchmarks to guide raters in their judgmental processes. The third column represents the calibration of the raters on the line that represents the latent variable. Column 3 provides a graphical display of the spread and location of raters from lenient to severe in their rating behaviors.

Column 4 represents the domains used to represent a framework for collecting observations that inform us regarding inferences of where persons are located on the latent variable. In the case of writing assessments, the domains include various aspects of the creation of meaningful text with appropriate attention to the mechanics of writing. In writing assessments, there are at least three rating formats used to define scoring guides for domains: holistic, analytic, and primary trait. Holistic formats ask the raters to provide an overall impression or judgment of an essay on a single domain (one rating), while analytic formats are used to obtain more detail from raters regarding the strengths and weaknesses of an essay in different domains (multiple ratings), such as meaning (organization and style) and mechanics (conventions and sentence formation). Primary trait scoring (Lloyd-Jones, 1977) is a type of analytic scoring that reflects the assignment of ratings based on the mode of discourse used for the writing tasks (multiple ratings). For example, student responses to a persuasive prompt would be rated with domains that include a judgment regarding how persuasive the writers were in their essays.

The researcher also decides on the response format to use to collect ratings. The structure of the rating scale can range from dichotomous ratings (0 = fail, 1 = pass) to rating scales (1 = inadequate, 2 = minimal, 3 = good, 4 = very good). The last column in the variable map represents the structure of the rating scale with the locations of the thresholds defining the empirical boundaries between the categories. An empirical boundary can be defined as the point on the line where the probability of getting a rating in the next higher category exceeds the probability of getting a rating in the adjacent lower category.

Rasch measurement models provide the psychometric theory for accomplishing this task of variable map construction. In essence, a variable map is a visual version of the operational definition of the latent variable or construct that includes the location on the scale of persons, raters, domains, and rating categories.

The scoring contexts listed in Table 9.3 can be used to illustrate variable maps within the context of rater-mediated assessments. Data from Gyagenda and Engelhard (2010) form the basis for these examples. Complete analyses of the Georgia Writing data are presented in the next chapter.

A simple scoring context for rater-mediated assessments includes multiple raters (at least two) using one domain with holistic scoring to rate student performance. The Many Facet model for this scoring context is

$$Ln \; [P_{nik} / P_{nik-1}] = \theta_n - \lambda_i - \tau_k$$

The variable map displaying results from rater assessments of student performances in this scoring context is shown in Figure 9.3. The first column is the logit scale (–10 to 10 logits). The next column gives the location of the persons on the variable map with low achieving students at the bottom and high achieving students at the top. The third column gives the location of three raters ranging from a lenient rater to a severe rater. The fourth column gives the location of one domain (meaning/organization) that is located at zero logits. Finally, the last column presents the ranges of expected ratings on the scale from 1 (inadequate) to 4 (very good). The cut points between these categories are the three thresholds demarcating the locations across adjacent category boundaries (1 to 2, 2 to 3, and 3 to 4). There is one less threshold than the number of categories with three thresholds in this example for the four rating categories.

Raters using analytic rubrics to assess students on multiple domains can also be modeled with the Many Facet Model. A single rater model is as follows:

$$Ln \; [P_{nik} / P_{nik-1}] = \theta_n - \delta_i - \tau_k$$

The variable map for this scoring context is shown in Figure 9.4. The variable map in Figure 9.4 is comparable to the map in Figure 9.3 with two differences: only one rater is represented on this variable map in Figure 9.4 (Rater 1), and the rater assessed students in multiple domains. Column 4 indicates that the mechanical aspects of writing (mechanics/conventions and mechanics/sentence formation are easier when compared to the creation of meaning (meaning organization and meaning/style).

Finally, the equation for multiple raters using multiple domains (analytic scoring) is:

$$Ln \; [P_{nmik} / P_{nmik-1}] = \theta_n - \lambda_m - \delta_i - \tau_k$$

The variable maps for this scoring context is shown in Figure 9.5. Again, this variable map is similar to the earlier maps shown in Figure 9.2 and 9.3 with the exception that Figure 9.5 includes the location of the raters on the variable map. Raters at the lower end of the scale are more lenient (Rater 15) as compared to raters who are located near the top of the variable map (Rater 9).

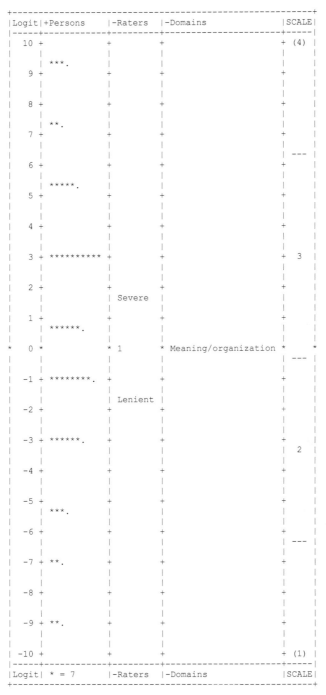

```
+--------------------------------------------------------------+
|Logit|+Persons    |-Raters  |-Domains            |SCALE|
|-----+-----------+---------+--------------------+-----|
|  10 +           +         +                    +  (4) |
|     |           |         |                    |      |
|     | ***.      |         |                    |      |
|   9 +           +         +                    +      |
|     |           |         |                    |      |
|     |           |         |                    |      |
|   8 +           +         +                    +      |
|     |           |         |                    |      |
|     | **.       |         |                    |      |
|   7 +           +         +                    +      |
|     |           |         |                    |      |
|     |           |         |                    | --- |
|   6 +           +         +                    +      |
|     |           |         |                    |      |
|     | *****.    |         |                    |      |
|   5 +           +         +                    +      |
|     |           |         |                    |      |
|     |           |         |                    |      |
|   4 +           +         +                    +      |
|     |           |         |                    |      |
|     |           |         |                    |      |
|   3 + ********** +         +                    +  3   |
|     |           |         |                    |      |
|     |           |         |                    |      |
|   2 +           +         +                    +      |
|     |           | Severe  |                    |      |
|     |           |         |                    |      |
|   1 +           +         +                    +      |
|     | ******.   |         |                    |      |
| *   0 *          * 1      * Meaning/organization *     *
|     |           |         |                    | --- |
|     |           |         |                    |      |
|  -1 + ********. +         +                    +      |
|     |           |         |                    |      |
|     |           | Lenient |                    |      |
|  -2 +           +         +                    +      |
|     |           |         |                    |      |
|     |           |         |                    |      |
|  -3 + ******.   +         +                    +      |
|     |           |         |                    |  2   |
|     |           |         |                    |      |
|  -4 +           +         +                    +      |
|     |           |         |                    |      |
|     |           |         |                    |      |
|  -5 +           +         +                    +      |
|     | ***.      |         |                    |      |
|     |           |         |                    |      |
|  -6 +           +         +                    + --- |
|     |           |         |                    |      |
|     |           |         |                    |      |
|  -7 + **.       +         +                    +      |
|     |           |         |                    |      |
|     |           |         |                    |      |
|  -8 +           +         +                    +      |
|     |           |         |                    |      |
|     |           |         |                    |      |
|  -9 + **.       +         +                    +      |
|     |           |         |                    |      |
|     |           |         |                    |      |
| -10 +           +         +                    +  (1) |
|-----+-----------+---------+--------------------+-----|
|Logit| * = 7      |-Raters  |-Domains            |SCALE|
+--------------------------------------------------------------+
```

Figure 9.3   Multiple raters using one domain (holistic scoring).

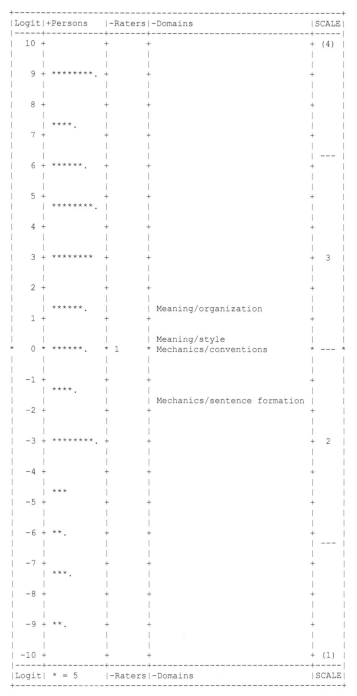

```
+-------------------------------------------------------------------+
|Logit|+Persons   |-Raters|-Domains                       | SCALE|
|-----+-----------+-------+-------------------------------+-----|
|  10 +           +       +                               + (4) |
|     |           |       |                               |     |
|     |           |       |                               |     |
|  9 + ********.  +       +                               +     |
|     |           |       |                               |     |
|     |           |       |                               |     |
|  8 +           +       +                               +     |
|     |           |       |                               |     |
|     | ****.     |       |                               |     |
|  7 +           +       +                               +     |
|     |           |       |                               |     |
|     |           |       |                               | --- |
|  6 + ******.   +       +                               +     |
|     |           |       |                               |     |
|     |           |       |                               |     |
|  5 +           +       +                               +     |
|     | ********. |       |                               |     |
|     |           |       |                               |     |
|  4 +           +       +                               +     |
|     |           |       |                               |     |
|     |           |       |                               |     |
|  3 + ********   +       +                               + 3   |
|     |           |       |                               |     |
|     |           |       |                               |     |
|  2 +           +       +                               +     |
|     |           |       |                               |     |
|     | ******.   |       | Meaning/organization          |     |
|  1 +           +       +                               +     |
|     |           |       |                               |     |
|     |           |       | Meaning/style                 |     |
*  0 * ******.    * 1    * Mechanics/conventions         * --- *
|     |           |       |                               |     |
| -1 +           +       +                               +     |
|     | ****.     |       |                               |     |
|     |           |       | Mechanics/sentence formation  |     |
| -2 +           +       +                               +     |
|     |           |       |                               |     |
|     |           |       |                               |     |
| -3 + ********.  +       +                               + 2   |
|     |           |       |                               |     |
|     |           |       |                               |     |
| -4 +           +       +                               +     |
|     |           |       |                               |     |
|     | ***       |       |                               |     |
| -5 +           +       +                               +     |
|     |           |       |                               |     |
|     |           |       |                               |     |
| -6 + **.        +       +                               +     |
|     |           |       |                               | --- |
|     |           |       |                               |     |
| -7 +           +       +                               +     |
|     | ***.      |       |                               |     |
|     |           |       |                               |     |
| -8 +           +       +                               +     |
|     |           |       |                               |     |
|     |           |       |                               |     |
| -9 + **.        +       +                               +     |
|     |           |       |                               |     |
|     |           |       |                               |     |
| -10 +           +       +                               + (1) |
|-----+-----------+-------+-------------------------------+-----|
|Logit| * = 5     |-Raters|-Domains                       | SCALE|
+-------------------------------------------------------------------+
```

Figure 9.4   One rater using multiple domains (analytic scoring).

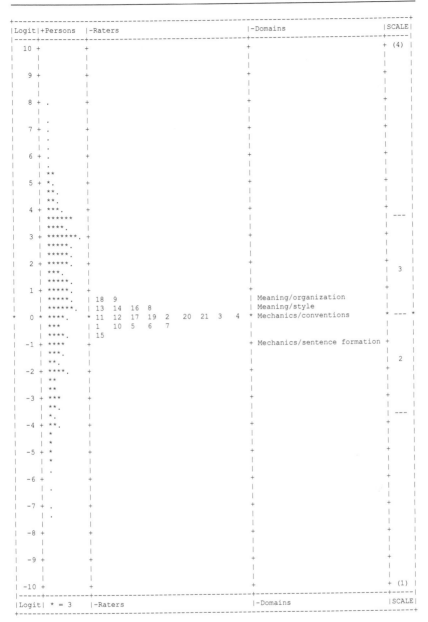

Figure 9.5   Multiple raters using multiple domains (analytic scoring).

Discussion and Summary

More than 30 years ago, Saal, Downey, and Lahey (1980) pointed out the extensive use of rating scales to communicate judgments. They also stressed the strong criticism and reservations that are connected with the use of rating scales:

... most of the reservations, regardless of how elegantly phrased, reflect fears that rating scale data are subjective (emphasizing, of course, the undesirable connotations of subjectivity), biased, and at worst, purposefully distorted. In the face of these often warranted misgivings, it is not surprising that psychologists and other professionals who rely on rating data have devoted much time and effort to the development of techniques and procedures for assessing the veracity and psychometric qualities of their judgmental measures. (p. 413)

This chapter illustrates the connections between a theory of judgmental processes (Brunswik, 1952; Hogarth, 1987) represented by a Lens Model, and a model-based approach to measurement theory using the Many Facets Model. The next chapter focuses on a variety of criteria that can be used to evaluate the psychometric quality of ratings obtained in rater-mediated assessments. A major theme of this chapter is that performance assessments and other assessments that require human raters introduce additional psychometric concerns over and above the typical issues encountered with multiple-choice items. Rater-mediated assessments provide a framework to clarify issues by explicitly recognizing that we are modeling of ratings based on human judgments, choices, interpretations, and decisions regarding the quality of a performance or product created by another person.

This chapter has highlighted several major points:

- Progress in performance assessment is reflected in the movement from ad hoc to theory and model-based methods and theories for examining the assessment processes.
- The judgmental and ecological aspects of judgmental processes have important examining the quality of the rating behavior of judges.
- A clearer understanding of these judgment processes can lead to strategies for examining and improving overall assessment processes.

The next chapter provides a detailed examination of methods for evaluating the quality of the judgments and ratings obtained from rater-mediated assessments.

Chapter 10

Evaluating the Quality of Rater-Mediated Assessments I

Indices of Rater Errors and Systematic Biases

Raters are human and they are therefore subject to all of the errors to which humankind must plead guilty.

(Guilford, 1936, p. 272)

This chapter describes methods for evaluating the quality of ratings obtained from rater-mediated assessments with illustrations based on the measurement of communicative competence in writing. Illustrative data analyses throughout this chapter are based on writing assessment using data described in Gyagenda and Engelhard (2010). The reader can generalize these methods to other areas of rater-mediated assessments. The research and topics covered in this chapter have implications for evaluating the quality of rating data in general. As with other areas of 20th-century measurement theory, the approaches to psychometrics and assessment within the context of rater-mediated assessments can be viewed in terms of two broad conceptual frameworks: test-score and scaling traditions.

The test-score tradition focuses on observed scores (observed ratings), and its primary goal is to decompose these observed ratings into true and error components (Observed score = true score + error score) with the results usually reported as variance components or reliability coefficients. The overarching goal is to determine the proportion of true score variance in the observed scores. Estimation of sources of error variance is a major focus of measurement approaches within the test-score tradition. Traditional approaches for examining rating quality within the test-score tradition have included rater agreement indices, inter-rater correlation coefficients, and various indices of rater reliability. In sorting through the traditional and commonly used methods, it is helpful to consider both the underlying issue being addressed by the statistical index, as well as the level of analysis. Table 10.1 summarizes three major categories (rater agreement, inter-rater correlation, and rater reliability) in terms of level of analysis (raters as individual or groups of raters. Statistical indices within each of these categories address aspects of the following questions:

- Do the raters agree with each other when assigning their ratings?
- Do the raters agree on the relative ordering of the persons?
- What is the ratio of true to total score variance in the ratings?

One of the most commonly used indices of rating quality within the test-score tradition is based on the agreement between raters regarding category usage. Rater agreement can be defined simply as the percentage of total ratings that categorize persons in the same manner. These agreement indices can be used to explore the agreement between each rater and every other rater when compared in a pairwise fashion, between each rater and all other raters, and agreement among the group of raters. Another common index of rating quality is based on the use of correlation coefficients (Pearson or Spearman). Inter-rater correlations explore whether or not the raters have ordered the person performances similarly. The third and final category of rating quality indices from a test-score tradition perspective relates to rater reliability. Rater reliability indices stress the importance of estimating the proportion of true to total score variance achieved in an assessment system. Generalizability Theory (Cronbach et al., 1972) and intra-class correlation coefficients (Shrout & Fleiss, 1979) are frequently used for this purpose.

Within the test-score tradition, some researchers prefer rater agreement indices as desirable indicators of rating quality, while other researchers prefer correlational indices as indicators of rating quality. The key point for current purposes is to recognize that rater agreement, rater correlations, and rater reliability indices reflect different underlying questions. See von Eye and Mun (2005) for a review of several other procedures that can be used to examine

Table 10.1 Test-Score Tradition: Rater Quality Indices by Level of Analysis and Underlying Questions

Categories	Level of Analysis	
	Individual Raters	Group of Raters
Rater agreement: Categorizing of persons	Does each rater agree with the ratings of another rater(s)?	Do the raters agree among themselves on the ratings?
Inter-rater correlation: Ordering of persons	Do the ratings of each rater correlate with ratings of another rater(s)?	Do the ratings of each rater correlate with ratings of the other raters?
Rater reliability: Estimating proportion of true score variance in observed person scores	How consistent are the ratings of each rater?	How consistent are the ratings for the assessment system?

rater agreement using observed ratings and test scores. In summary, rating quality indices within the test-score tradition stress:

1. rater agreement indices as that represent consensus among raters on the placement of persons in categories,
2. correlational indices for exploring coherent orderings of persons by raters, and
3. rater reliability indices that indicate the ratios of true score to total score variance in the observed ratings.

These indices can address questions related to individual raters and groups of raters as shown in Table 10.1.

The scaling tradition provides another theoretical framework for analyzing ratings. As pointed out repeatedly in this volume, the scaling tradition is a useful framework for examining whether or not invariant measurement has been achieved. The scaling tradition includes the idea of a variable map with the general goal of mapping facets of the rater-mediated assessment system onto an underlying latent variable. Measurement models in the scaling tradition, such as Rasch models for rating scale data, focus on estimating the locations of persons, raters, and domains on a variable map that represents the underlying construct.[1] Variable maps provide the organizing schema for evaluating the quality of rater-mediated assessments. Variable maps are an essential feature of invariant measurement.

The rest of this chapter focuses on the rater-mediated assessments as viewed through the lens of one particular scaling model: the Many Facet Model (Linacre, 1989). The specific topics addressed are related to Rasch-based methods for addressing psychometric issues related to rater errors and other systematic biases that arise in rater-mediated assessments.

Rater Errors and Systematic Biases

Traditional indices of rating quality tend to view errors as chance variations that are inadvertently introduced into the rater-mediated assessment system. Some researchers have suggested that there may also be systematic errors and biases related to construct-irrelevant aspects of rater behaviors and judgments (Hoyt, 2000; Hoyt & Kerns, 1999). For example, early work on the halo error by Thorndike (1920) identified raters that were not able to rate analytically

---

1　The use of Rasch measurement for rater-mediated assessments was introduced by Linacre (1989). The estimation procedures and model-data fit indices are implemented in the Facets computer program (Linacre, 2007). Mike Linacre completed his dissertation under the direction of Professor Ben Wright at the University of Chicago.

because of an overall impression or holistic judgment of a person that was either unreasonable positive (halo effect) or negative (pitchfork effect). There have been a variety of rater error indices that have been proposed for examining rater biases and other sources of systematic imprecision in rater-mediated assessment. Table 10.2 describes several rater errors by level of analysis and the underlying questions related to each error.

The four most commonly identified rater errors are severity/leniency, halo error, central tendency (response sets) and score range restriction (Saal,

Table 10.2 Description of Rater Errors by Level of Analysis and Underlying Questions

Definitions	Level of Analysis	
	Individual Raters	*Group of Raters*
Rater Severity/Leniency: The tendency on the part of raters to consistently provide higher or lower ratings than warranted by person performances.	How severe is each rater? Where is the rater located on the variable map?	Are the differences in rater severity significant? Can the raters be considered invariant and exchangeable?
Halo error: Rater fails to distinguish between conceptually distinct and independent aspects of person performances.	Is the rater distinguishing between conceptually distinct and independent domains?	Are the raters distinguishing among the domains?
Response sets (e.g., central tendency): Rater interprets and uses rating scale categories in an idiosyncratic fashion. Rater over uses middle categories of rating scale when not warranted by person performance.	Is the rater using the rating scales as intended?	Are the raters using the rating scales as intended?
Score Range Restriction: Raters do not discriminate between persons on the latent variable.	How well did each rater discriminate among the different persons?	Did the assessment system lead to the identification of meaningful individual differences among persons?
Interaction effects: Facets in the measurement model are not additive.	Is the rater interpreting and using the other facets in the model as designed?	Are the facets invariant across raters?
Differential facet functioning (DFF): Ratings are a function of construct-irrelevant components.	Are the ratings of each rater invariant over construct-irrelevant components?	Are the raters invariant over construct-irrelevant components for the overall assessment system?

Downey, & Lahey, 1980). Each of these rater errors is briefly described in Table 10.2. There is a hodgepodge of operational definitions and statistical indicators of these rater errors that have been proposed for evaluating and monitoring raters to detect these four categories of response bias (Myford & Wolfe, 2004).

The ad hoc and atheoretical nature of the research on rater errors has led some researchers to conclude that "rater error measures should be abandoned" (Murphy & Cleveland, 1995, p. 285). Specifically, Murphy and Cleveland (1995) argued that current rater error measures are not useful criteria for evaluating performance ratings because (a) the unit of analysis is defined incorrectly, and (b) the distribution assumptions regarding persons are frequently not met or are unreasonable. Both of these concerns are correct and reflect the fact that current indices of rater errors are based on the test-score tradition, and this research tradition typically defines the unit of analysis in terms of groups rather than individual raters. Indices based in the test-score tradition also yield sample dependent results that are not invariant across persons and depend upon various distributional assumptions that may or may not be met with a particular group of persons. Although Murphy and Cleveland (1995) are correct in their criticism of current rater error indices, their call for the abandonment of rater error indices in general is premature. The Many Facet (MF) model provides a theoretically sound and conceptually clear way of defining a family of rater errors. It provides a focus on the individual rater as the unit of analysis and addresses issues of systematic biases across groups of raters. The MF model also provides the opportunity to achieve invariant measurement that does not depend on the distributional vagaries of the particular sample of persons used to calibrate the assessment system.

Table 10.2 defines the commonly examined rater errors: rater severity/leniency, halo error, response sets (e.g., central tendency) and range restriction from the perspective of the MF model. In addition to rater errors and systematic biases, two other categories of rater errors are included: interaction effects and differential facet functioning. The underlying questions for individual raters and the rater group are also presented in Table 10.2. MF model indices can be used to address each of these questions. The MF model indices represent a model-based approach that address traditional concerns regarding rater errors, explores additional questions regarding systematic response biases not traditionally considered, and adds to the methodological tool box of the researchers exploring the quality of ratings obtained within the context of rater-mediated assessments.

The writing assessment data used in this chapter (Gyagenda & Engelhard, 2010) is analyzed with a Many Facet model for multiple raters using multiple domains (analytic scoring) with a four-category rating scale:

$$\text{Ln}\,[P_{nmik}\,/\,P_{nmik-1}] = \theta_n - \lambda_m - \delta_i - \tau_k \qquad [1]$$

where

P_{nmik} = probability of person n being rated k on domain i by rater m,
P_{nmik-1} = probability of person n being rated k-1 on domain i by rater m,
θ_n = judged location of person n,
λ_m = severity of rater m,
δ_j = judged difficulty of domain i, and
τ_k = judged difficulty of rating category k relative to category k–1.

The rating category coefficient, τ_k, is not generally considered a facet in the model. Figure 10.1 provides the lens model for a writing assessment that represents Equation 1.

This model adds potential construct-irrelevant components to the model that was introduced in Chapter 9. The dependent variable in the model is the observed ratings. The major facets that define the intervening variables used to make the latent variable (writing competence) observable are rater severity and two cues: domains and rating scale. The third facet that represents the target or object of measurement is writing competence (person). The structure of the rating scale (e.g., number of rating categories) also plays a fundamental role in defining the observed ratings. Although the structure of the rating scale is not explicitly considered a facet in the model, it is an important intervening component from the perspective of a lens model for rater-mediated assessments.

The model in Figure 10.1 also explicitly introduces a set of potential construct-irrelevant sources of variance. There are at least two potential groups of

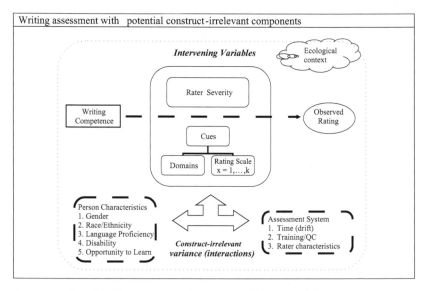

Figure 10.1 Lens Models for Writing Assessments (Observed ratings).

variables: person characteristics and characteristics of the assessment system. The key idea is that these construct-irrelevant variables influence the how the raters are using cues (domains and rating scale) that may interfere with the quality of the ratings. For example, raters may interpret the domains differentially when used to assign ratings to boys and girls. The interaction between gender and domain can be viewed as a type of differential item functioning that has been extensively studied within the context of multiple-choice items (Zumbo, 1999). In addition to the person characteristics that may interact with the intervening variables, it is also possible that certain aspects of the assessment system may also provide sources of construct-irrelevant variation. For example, raters may change their severity over time during the scoring session. This rater drift can be monitored, and it should be systematically studied so that persons who are rated at different time points are not unduly affected by variation in rater severity or leniency (Myford & Wolfe, 2009; Wolfe, Myford, Engelhard, & Manalo, 2007).

Once the parameters of the model in Equation 1 are estimated using standard numerical methods, such as those implemented in the Facets computer program (Linacre 2007), model-data fit issues can be examined in a variety of ways. In order to attain invariant measurement, the model must fit the data; lack of model-data fit indicates that the requirements of invariant measurement have not been met. Useful indices of rating quality can be obtained by a detailed examination of the standardized residuals calculated as

$$Z_{ni} = (x_{ni} - E_{ni}) / [\sum_{k=1}^{m} (k - E_{ni})^2 P_{nik}]^{1/2} \qquad [2]$$

where

$$E_{ni} = \sum_{k=1}^{m} k P_{nik} \qquad [3]$$

and xnmi is the observed rating for person n from rater m on domain i. The standardized residuals, Znmi, can be summarized over different facets and different elements within a facet in order to provide indices of model-data fit. These residuals are typically summarized as mean square error statistics called Outfit and Infit statistics. For example, the mean square error statistics for the rater facet can be calculated as follows:

$$Outfit_m = \frac{\sum_{n=1}^{N} \sum_{i=1}^{I} Z_{nmi}^2}{NI} \qquad [4]$$

where m is the rater index, n is the person index and i is the domain index. The Outfit statistics are unweighted mean squared residual statistics that are particularly sensitive to outlying unexpected ratings. A weighted version of these mean squared residual statistics called Infit statistics can also be calculated. These Infit statistics are less sensitive to outlying unexpected ratings. The expected value of both of these fit statistics is 1.0 when the model fits the data with a standard deviation of .20. Mean square error statistics with values less than 1.0 indicate less variability in the ratings than expected, while values greater than 1.0 indicate more variability than expected. Wright and Masters (1982) provide a lucid description and illustration of Infit and Outfit statistics. The substantive interpretation of these mean square error statistics varies depending on the facet. The exact sampling distribution of these fit statistics is not known, and there are no exact tests of statistical significance; various rules of thumb have been proposed for interpreting these values that are useful in practice. For example, some rules of thumb suggest Infit and Outfit values between .80 and 1.20 for multiple-choice items, and values between .60 and 1.5 for constructed-response items depending on the context of the assessment.

Another useful statistic is the reliability of separation index. This index provides information about how well the elements or levels within a facet are separated in order to reliably define the facet. For the person facet, this index is analogous to traditional indices of reliability, such as Cronbach's coefficient alpha and KR20, in the sense that it reflects an estimate of the ratio of true score to observed score variance. It can be calculated as

$$R = (SD^2 - MSE) / SD^2, \qquad [5]$$

where SD2 is the observed variance of element difficulties for a facet on the latent variable scale in logits and MSE is the mean square calibration error estimated as the mean of the calibration error variances (squares of the standard errors) for each element within a facet. Andrich (1982) provides a detailed derivation of this reliability of separation index. An approximate chi-square statistic for judging the statistical significance of the differences between elements within a facet can also be calculated; this statistic is analogous to the homogeneity test statistic Q described by Hedges and Olkin (1985).

Illustrative Data Analyses

The next three sections focus on each of the three facets from a Many Facets analysis of the writing data from Gyagenda and Engelhard (2010). Before discussing each facet in turn, it is useful to examine the overall functioning of the Many Facet model for these data. Table 10.3 gives the overall summary statistics for the rater, domain and person facets of the model from the Facets computer program. There are several things to note in this summary table. First of all, the rater facet is centered with a mean of zero (SD = .34), and the domain facets is also centered at zero (SD = .66). Since the object of measurement is persons, the person facet is not centered (M = .80, SD = 2.84). The

Table 10.3 Summary Statistics for Raters, Domains, and Persons

	Raters	Domains	Persons
Measure			
Mean	.00	00	.80
SD	.34	.66	2.84
N	21	4	365
Outfit			
Mean	.98	.98	.98
SD	.19	.05	.26
Infit			
Mean	.97	.97	.98
SD	.17	.05	.22
Separation statistic			
Reliability of separation	.98	.99	.99
Chi-square	846.7*	2543.8*	47417.4*
(df)	(20)	(3)	(364)

* $p < .05$

convention in the Many Facet model is to center all of the facets except the one that represents the object of measurement. This provides a stable frame of reference for interpreting the locations of raters, domains, and persons on the variable map. The summary fit statistics (Infit and Outfit) are close to the expected values of 1.00 with a standard deviation of .20 indicating fairly good model-data fit. In addition to the summary statistics, the rating scale structure for these data was examined. Table 10.4 gives the rating category usage by the 21 raters. Based on the guidelines given in Chapter 9, the rating scale appears to be working as intended (i.e., as a four-category scale), with raters assigning ratings in all four categories.

Figure 10.2 presents the category characteristic and expected score function for these data. Panel A shows the category characteristic function, and

Table 10.4 Rating Scale Structure

Rating	Usage	Average Measure	Expected Measure	Outfit	Thresholds	Labels
1	10%	-3.84	-3.91	1.00	Low	Inadequate
2	29%	-1.13	-1.06	1.00	-3.52	Minimal
3	39%	1.72	1.69	1.00	.07	Good
4	21%	4.03	4.01	1.00	3.45	Very good

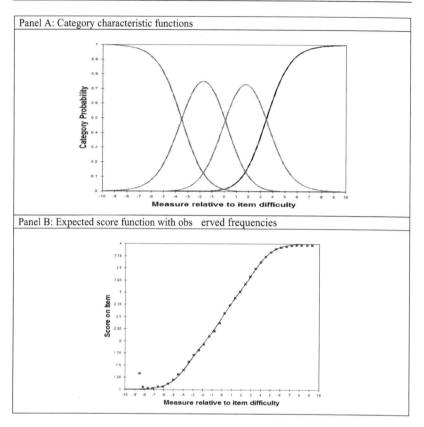

Panel A: Category characteristic functions

Panel B: Expected score function with obs   erved frequencies

Figure 10.2 Category characteristic and expected score functions for the rating scale.

as presented in Table 10.4 these curves indicate that the rating scale is working very well. Panel B shows the expected score function with the observed frequencies included as a visual display of model-data fit. The expected score function is also called a test characteristic curve in item response theory. The expected score function represents the connection between the theta scale on the x-axis, and the expected score (or sometimes percentage of total available score points) on the y-axis. Again, good agreement between the model and the data is indicated by an inspection of Panel B.

I. Rater Facet

Table 10.5 presents 10 indices that provide evidence regarding the quality of ratings for the rater facet using the Many Facet model. Evidence regarding rater severity/leniency errors can be detected by using the first five statistical indices in Table 10.5. Figure 10.3 presents the variable map for 21 raters using

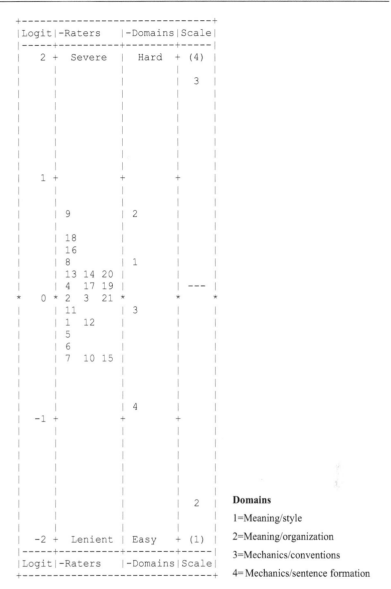

```
+-------------------------------+
|Logit|-Raters    |-Domains|Scale|
|-----+-----------+--------+-----|
|  2 +    Severe   |  Hard  + (4) |
|     |            |        |     |
|     |            |        |   3 |
|     |            |        |     |
|     |            |        |     |
|     |            |        |     |
|     |            |        |     |
|     |            |        |     |
|     |            |        |     |
|  1 +            +        +     |
|     |            |        |     |
|     |            |        |     |
|     | 9          | 2      |     |
|     |            |        |     |
|     | 18         |        |     |
|     | 16         |        |     |
|     | 8          | 1      |     |
|     | 13 14 20   |        |     |
|     | 4  17 19   |        | --- |
*  0 * 2  3  21  *        *     *
|     | 11         | 3      |     |
|     | 1  12      |        |     |
|     | 5          |        |     |
|     | 6          |        |     |
|     | 7  10 15   |        |     |
|     |            |        |     |
|     |            |        |     |
|     |            | 4      |     |
| -1 +            +        +     |
|     |            |        |     |
|     |            |        |     |
|     |            |        |     |
|     |            |        |     |
|     |            |        |     |
|     |            |        |   2 |
|     |            |        |     |
|     |            |        |     |
| -2 +   Lenient  |  Easy  + (1) |
|-----+-----------+--------+-----|
|Logit|-Raters    |-Domains|Scale|
+-------------------------------+
```

Domains

1=Meaning/style

2=Meaning/organization

3=Mechanics/conventions

4=Mechanics/sentence formation

Figure 10.3 Variable map for raters, domains and rating scale (person facet not included).

four domains with a four-category rating scale. In the variable map, the scale on the left-hand side of the figure is in logits. An examination of Figure 10.3 shows how the raters are distributed on the variable map. A version of this map was presented in Chapter 9 (Figure 9.5) with the person facet included.

Table 10.5 Scaling Tradition: Statistical Indices and Graphical Displays of Rating
Quality Based on the Many Facet Model (Raters, Domains, and Persons)

Indices and Displays	*1. Rater Facet*	*2. Domain Facet*	*3. Person Facet*
1. Variable map	Where are the raters located on the latent variable or construct being measured?	Where are the domains located on the latent variable or construct being measured?	Where are the persons located on the latent variable or construct being measured?
2. Calibration and location of elements within facet	What is the location of each rater (severity/leniency)?	What is the judged difficulty of each domain?	What is the judged location on the latent variable of each person?
3. Standard errors for each element	How precisely has each rater been calibrated?	How precisely has each domain been calibrated?	How precisely has each person been calibrated?
4. Reliability of separation	How spread out are the rater severities? Are the raters exchangeable?	How spread out are the domain difficulties? Are the raters distinguishing among the domains?	How spread out are the judged person locations?
5. Chi-square statistic	Are the overall differences between the raters statistically significant?	Are the overall differences between the domains statistically significant?	Are the overall differences between the persons statistically significant?
6. Infit and Outfit Statistics (Mean square error)	How consistently has each rater interpreted the domains and categories across persons?	How consistently has each domain been interpreted and used by the raters?	How consistently has person performance been interpreted by the raters?
7. Standardized residuals	How different is each observed rating from its expected value?	How different is each observed rating from its expected value?	How different is each observed rating from its expected value?
8. Quality control charts, figures and tables (displays of residuals)	What individual ratings appear to be higher or lower than expected based on the model?	What individual ratings appear to be higher or lower than expected based on the model?	What individual ratings appear to be higher or lower than expected based on the model?
9. Interaction effects	Are there significant interaction effects between raters and other facets?	Are there significant interaction effects between domains and other facets?	Are there significant interaction effects between persons and other facets?

Indices and Displays	1. Rater Facet	2. Domain Facet	3. Person Facet
10. Differential facet functioning	Are the rater severities invariant across subgroups?	Are the judged domain difficulties invariant across subgroups?	Are the judged person locations invariant across raters?

The results from the calibration of the raters are shown in Table 10.6. The raters range in severity from Rater 15 who is the most lenient (–.55 logits) to Rater 9 who is the most severe (.75 logits). The overall differences between raters as a group is summarized as a reliability of rater separation index and the chi-square statistic to estimate statistical significance as seen in Table 10.3. The overall differences between raters shown in Figure 10.3 and Table 10.6 are statistically significant [$\chi^2(20) = 846.7$, p < .05] with a high reliability

Table 10.6 Calibration of Rater Facet

Raters	Mean Rating	Measure (logits)	S.E.	Infit	Outfit	Slope	N
9	2.52	0.75	0.05	0.76	0.73	1.27	365
18	2.58	0.50	0.05	1.11	1.28	0.86	365
16	2.61	0.41	0.05	0.97	1.06	1.00	365
8	2.65	0.27	0.05	0.93	0.91	1.09	365
13	2.67	0.18	0.05	1.00	0.99	0.99	365
14	2.67	0.17	0.05	1.02	1.06	0.99	365
20	2.68	0.15	0.05	1.00	1.01	1.00	365
17	2.69	0.11	0.05	0.81	0.80	1.21	365
4	2.69	0.10	0.05	0.81	0.79	1.21	365
19	2.70	0.07	0.05	1.24	1.21	0.73	365
3	2.72	-0.01	0.05	0.97	1.05	1.02	365
2	2.72	-0.02	0.05	0.80	0.78	1.22	365
21	2.73	-0.04	0.05	1.26	1.21	0.73	365
11	2.73	-0.08	0.05	0.82	0.80	1.20	365
12	2.76	-0.17	0.05	0.87	0.89	1.13	365
1	2.77	-0.19	0.05	0.58	0.54	1.49	365
5	2.78	-0.26	0.05	1.17	1.16	0.81	365
6	2.83	-0.44	0.05	0.97	0.98	1.04	365
10	2.84	-0.48	0.05	1.05	1.07	0.94	365
7	2.84	-0.49	0.05	1.21	1.22	0.77	365
15	2.86	-0.55	0.05	1.00	1.10	0.95	365

Note. Raters 18 and 20 have the lowest and highest Outfit statistics respectively.

of separation index (R = .98). The reliability of separation index for raters provides overall information regarding variability in raters, and it can be used as an omnibus descriptive index for rater effects at the group level.

Table 10.6 also includes a summary of the standardized residuals for each rater in terms of the mean square fit statistics (Infit and Outfit statistics). Rater 1 has the smallest Outfit statistic (Outfit = .54), while Rater 18 has the largest outfit statistic (Outfit = 1.28). Raters with low mean square fit statistics tend have muted ratings that suggest a halo error. For example, Rater 1 had rated 37.8% of the essays with uniform rating patterns (e.g., 1111, 22222, 33333, and 4444). These raters may be rating holistically rather than differentiating between the persons when assigning ratings for the four domains. As shown in Table 10.5, the Infit and Outfit statistics can be used to explore halo and other types of response sets (e.g., restriction of range) exhibited in the ratings.

Information regarding muted and noisy rating patterns can be presented using quality control charts. The individual observed ratings with standard-ized residuals less than –2.00 and greater than +2.00 can be flagged for further examination. Quality control charts for Rater 18 (Outfit = 1.28, noisy rating pattern) and Rater 1 (Outfit = .54, muted rating pattern) are shown in Figure 10.4. Panel A shows Rater 18 with some ratings outside of the range of –2.00

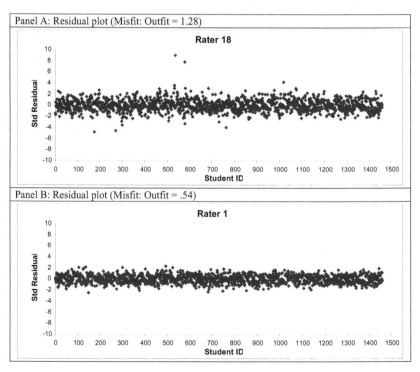

Figure 10.4   Quality control charts: Residual plots for Raters 18 and 1.

to +2.00, while Panel B shows Rater 1 with almost all of the ratings within this range.

Although interaction effects can be detected by analyzing the standardized residuals, it is also useful for monitoring raters to consider interaction effects explicitly. For example, the model for a three-facet assessment system (persons, raters, domains) with a two-way interaction effect between rater and domain (rater x domain) can be written as follows:

$$Ln\ [P_{nmik} / P_{nmik-1}] = \theta_n - \lambda_m - \delta_i - \lambda_m\ \delta_i - \tau_k \qquad [2]$$

This model can be used to explore whether or not the relative difficulties of the domains are invariant over raters. In other words, are the raters using and interpreting the domains in a consistent and comparable fashion. The Facets computer program (Linacre, 2007) can be used to calculate these interaction effects.

Panel A in Figure 10.5 illustrates the interaction effect between raters and domains. Thisdisplay suggests that raters may interpret the domains differently. The judgmental ordering of the domains is not invariant across all of the raters when the lines cross indicating an interaction effect. For example, Rater 1 orders the domains as follows:

1. Meaning/organization
2. Meaning/style
3. Mechanics/sentence formation
4. *Mechanics/conventions*

The order of the domains for Raters 11 and 15 are different with mechanics/conventions at the top:

1. **Mechanics/conventions**
2. Meaning/organization
3. Meaning/style
4. Mechanics/sentence formation

The interpretation of the cues reflected in the domains and used by these different raters define the ratings assigned by these raters. If the ratings are not invariant across the four domains used to define writing, then the judged quality of the essays do not have the same meaning across raters.

Differential facet functioning (DFF) is numerically equivalent to observations of interaction effects, but it is listed separately in Table 10.5 to highlight that the interactions being explored are potential construct-irrelevant components related to person characteristics and assessment system characteristics as shown in Figure 10.1. For example, the model for a three-facet assessment

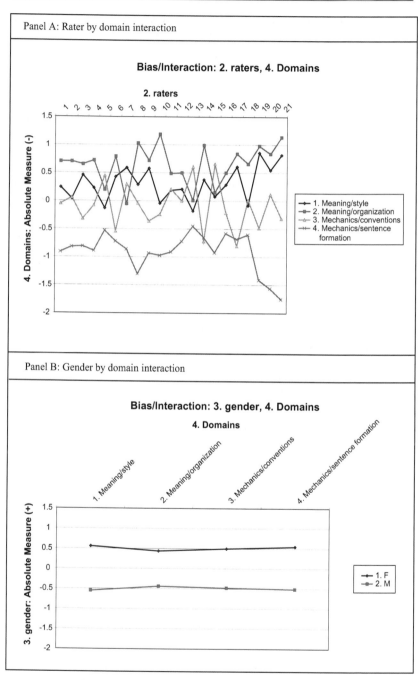

Figure 10.5 Interaction plots for raters by domains and gender by domains.

system (persons, raters, domains) with a fourth explanatory facet (gender) added to explore DFF can be written as follows:

$$Ln\ [P_{nmijk} / P_{nmijk-1}] = \theta_n - \lambda_m - \delta_i - \gamma_j - \delta_i\gamma_j - \tau_k$$

In this case the focus is on whether or not the gender facet, γ_j, interacts with the domain facet, δ_i. If there are significant interaction effects, $\delta_i\gamma_j$, then this would provide evidence that the severities of the raters were not invariant over gender groups. In other words, some raters are rating either girls or boys more harshly than justified by their performance. Panel B in Figure 10.5 displays the interaction effect between domain and gender. In this case, the data suggests that there is not an interaction effect, and that girls tend to have higher rating than boys across all four domains.

2. Domain Facet

Turning now to the domain facet, the same set of statistical indices and graphical displays used to examine the rater facet can also be used to evaluate the functioning of the domains. The domain specific interpretations and questions underlying the MF model indices are given in Table 10.5. Similar information is provided by these indices for both domains and raters, although the substantive questions being address by the indices and displays vary somewhat for the domain facet. It should be stressed here that the domain difficulties and other domain-based indices are also providing information regarding how the raters are interpreting and using the rater-mediated assessment system. Domain difficulty is defined by the judgments and interpretations of the raters. The results from the calibration of the domains are summarized in Table 10.7. Figure 10.3 shows that the analytic domains range from being relatively easy (−.89 logits, 4. mechanics/sentence formation domain) to being relatively hard (.65 logits, 2. Meaning/organization domain). As shown in Table 10.3, the overall differences between the domain difficulties are statistically significant $\chi^2(3) = 2543.8$, p < .05 with a high reliability of separation index (R = .99). This provides support for the inference that the raters are adequately distinguishing between the domains as intended by the test developers. Based on the Outfit and Infit statistics, there is no evidence that the raters are interpreting the domains in an inconsistent fashion because all of the mean square statistics are between .8 and 1.2.

3. Person Facet

The object of measurement for the writing assessment system is the person. The goal is to develop a measure to represent writing competence for each person, and to display the location of each person on the variable map representing this construct. The summary statistics are presented in Table 10.3.

Table 10.7 Domains of Writing

Domains	Mean	Measure	S.E.	Infit	Outfit
Meaning/ organization	2.54	0.65	0.02	0.97	0.99
Meaning/style	2.64	0.31	0.02	1.02	1.05
Mechanics/ conventions	2.74	-0.07	0.02	0.91	0.93
Mechanics/ sentence formation	2.94	-0.89	0.02	0.98	0.97

The estimates of writing competence (N = 365) ranged from –7.43 to 8.05 logits (M =.80, SD =2.84). The overall differences between the students were statistically significant [$\chi^2(364)$ = 47417.4, p < .05] with a high reliability of separation index (R = .99). In terms of the rater errors listed in Table 10.2, these analyses for the person facet suggest that score range restriction was not an issue for this group of raters.

Diagnostic information regarding the raters is also available in the Infit and Outfit statistics from the 375 student essays. Students with higher Infit and Outfit statistics exhibit noisy rating patterns, while students with lower Infit and Outfit statistics tend to have muted rating patterns. Noisy rating patterns have a high number of unexpected ratings, while muted ratings patterns tend to exhibit uniform ratings. Both of these patterns may reflect idiosyncratic ratings or response sets, such as central tendency or halo, on the part of the raters when they assign ratings to these essays. Table 10.8 provides a quality control table for Person 675.

Person 675 has a noisy rating pattern (INFIT = 1.80, OUTFIT = 1.85). This person received unexpectedly high ratings on the meaning/organization domain from Raters 11 and 19, and unexpectedly low ratings from Raters 20 and 21. The essays of this person should be flagged and examined to determine whether or not there are any reasons to rescore this essay. Quality control charts can also be created for persons that mirror Figure 10.4.

Rater Invariant Measurement

The goal of rater-invariant person measurement is to develop an assessment system that can be used to measure a person's location on a latent variable that is not dependent on the particular raters who happen to rate the person. In order to illustrate this idea, a variable map is presented in Figure 10.6. This is a variable map for Person A with a location on the latent variable at zero (θ_A = 0.00). There are three sets of raters (Sets 1, 2, and 3) with each set composed of four raters who vary in severity or location on the latent variable. For example,

Table 10.8 Ratings for Person 675 with Unexpected Rating Patterns (Infit=1.80, Outfit 1.81)

Index	Person	Rater	Domain	Observed Rating	Expected Rating	Residual	Standardized Residual (Z)
1	675	1	Meaning/organization	3	2.39	0.61	1.10
2	675	10	Meaning/organization	2	2.48	-0.48	-0.86
3	675	11	Meaning/organization	4	2.36	1.64	3.00
4	675	12	Meaning/organization	3	2.39	0.61	1.12
5	675	13	Meaning/organization	2	2.28	-0.28	-0.53
6	675	14	Meaning/organization	3	2.29	0.71	1.33
7	675	15	Meaning/organization	3	2.50	0.50	0.89
8	675	16	Meaning/organization	3	2.22	0.78	1.49
9	675	17	Meaning/organization	3	2.30	0.70	1.29
10	675	18	Meaning/organization	3	2.19	0.81	1.55
11	675	19	Meaning/organization	4	2.32	1.68	3.11
12	675	2	Meaning/organization	3	2.34	0.66	1.21
13	675	20	Meaning/organization	1	2.29	-1.29	-2.40
14	675	21	Meaning/organization	1	2.35	-1.35	-2.47
15	675	3	Meaning/organization	2	2.34	-0.34	-0.62
16	675	4	Meaning/organization	3	2.31	0.69	1.28
17	675	5	Meaning/organization	3	2.41	0.59	1.06
18	675	6	Meaning/organization	3	2.47	0.53	0.95
19	675	7	Meaning/organization	3	2.48	0.52	0.93
20	675	8	Meaning/organization	3	2.26	0.74	1.39
21	675	9	Meaning/organization	3	2.13	0.87	1.70

Rater Set 1 is composed of four raters with the following severities: λ_{12} = -2.00, λ_{14} = -.50, λ_{15} = .50 and λ_{17} = 1.50. Based on the Rasch model, persons with locations above the rater severity are expected to receive a particular rating. In Figure 10.6, Column 1 represents the underlying latent variable on the logit scale, Columns 2 to 4 represent the rater locations within rater sets 1, 2, and 3. Column 5 shows the location of the person on the scale, while the next three columns indicate the ratings that Person A received from raters in each of the three rater sets. It should be clear in this figure that if the person is rated as expected based on the model, then Person A's summed ratings from Rater Set 1 is 12 (Mean of 3.0 on four-category rating scale). By contrast, the summed ratings from Rater Set 2 is 14 (Mean of 3.5 on four-category rating scale), and on the summed ratings from Rater Set 3 is 10 (Mean of 2.5 on four-category rating scale). This example demonstrates how summed ratings are not invariant over different subsets of raters who vary in severity. As was the

Logit Scale	Rater Sets			Person A	Observed Ratings			Ratings (Thresholds)
	Set 1 (Fair)	Set 2 (Easy)	Set 3 (Hard)	Theta	Set 1 (Fair)	Set 2 (Easy)	Set 3 (Hard	
5.00								(1)
4.00								
3.00			λ_{38}				2	2
2.00			λ_{37}		2			
	λ_{17}						2	
1.00			λ_{36}				3	
	λ_{15}	λ_{25}			3	3		
.00				θ_A= .00				3
	λ_{14}				3			
-1.00		λ_{23}	λ_{33}			3	3	
-2.00	λ_{12}	λ_{22}			4	4		
-3.00		λ_{21}				4		
-4.00								(4)
-5.00								
Mean:	.00	-1.5	1.5	Sum:	12	14	10	

Note. Person location on latent variable is fixed (θ_A = .00). Responses and sum scores are dependent on the particular rater severities for rater sets (Sets 1, 2 and 3). Sum scores are not invariant over subsets of raters.

Figure 10.6 Variable Map for Person A: Rater-invariant person measurement (θ_A = .00).

case with item sets in Chapter 2, it is possible to adjust for rater severity differences within the context of Rasch measurement theory in order to preserve the invariant location of Person A on the latent variable scale.

This chapter introduced a family of rater error indices that reflect a potential lack of invariance in various aspects of rater-mediated assessment systems. This section also included examples from large-scale writing assessments to illustrate these psychometric indices of rater errors. The next section introduces a family of accuracy indices that focus on a different aspect of the quality of ratings obtained from rater-mediated assessments.

Discussion and Summary

The models and methods described in this chapter and the previous one provide a strong theoretical basis for examining rater judgments. These models provide a solid framework for assessment systems based on human judgments. This chapter presented a set of procedures based on the Many Facet model (Linacre, 1989) that can be used to evaluate and monitor raters within the context of large-scale performance assessments. The Many Facet model represents a model-based approach to assessment (Embretson, 2010) that meets the requirements of invariant measurement (Engelhard, 1994) and reflects the new rules of measurement (Embretson, 1996). It is essential that rater-mediated assessments move from ad hoc procedures to model-based indices of rating quality. The indices of rater errors described in this chapter are based on the theoretical requirements of invariant measurement and the application of Rasch measurement theory to detect whether or not invariant measurement has been realized.

Some of the major advantages of the Many Facet (MF) model described in this chapter are as follows (Engelhard, 2002):

- The MF model is a scaling model that employs a logistic transformation to convert qualitative ratings into linear measures. The observed ratings are on an ordinal scale, while the estimates of person ability on the construct are on a linear scale. If the degree of model-data fit is high, then the ability measures have equal-interval properties.
- The MF model provides an explicit and model-based approach for examining multiple facets encountered in performance assessment systems. A sound theoretical framework is provided for adjusting for differences in rater severity. If the degree of model-data fit is high, then invariant estimates of person ability can be obtained across different subsets of raters. Statistical adjustments for rater severity differences can only be justified when model-data fit is good. These invariant estimates improve the objectivity and fairness of the overall assessment system.

- If model-data fit is good, then invariant calibration of the rater-mediated assessment and rater-invariant measurement is possible. Various statistical indices and graphical displays are available based on the MF model to explore sources of misfit and identify potential problems.

In summary, the MF model offers an approach for addressing a variety of issues that may be encountered in rater-mediated performance assessments. In order to develop clear and unambiguous measures of variables based on rater-mediated assessments, it is essential that the various facets of the model be invariant across raters and other construct-irrelevant components. As pointed out in the opening quote, it is important to remember that there are limits on our efforts: "Raters are human and they are therefore subject to all the errors to which humankind must plead guilty" (Guilford, 1936, p. 272). The approach for identifying, evaluating, and monitoring rater errors based on the MF model can decrease some response biases, but it is unlikely any assessment system can totally eliminate response biases because raters are human. The next chapter introduces direct indices of rating quality based on an examination of rater accuracy.

Chapter 11

Evaluating the Quality
of Rater-Mediated Assessments II

Indices of Rater Accuracy

A general framework for conceptualizing rater-mediated assessments based on a lens model was described in Chapter 9. Chapter 10 introduced a family of indices that can be used to examine the quality of ratings viewed as rater errors and systematic biases. The current chapter continues the discussion of indices that can be used for evaluating rating quality. If the potential rater error and biases indices described in Chapter 10 are considered *indirect measures* of rating quality, then the rater accuracy indices described in this chapter offer *direct measures* for exploring how closely a set of observed ratings match a set of known or true ratings. In essence, the rater accuracy model defines the latent variable as accuracy, and the purpose of the assessment is to evaluate facets of rater accuracy in a manner comparable to the ways in which other Rasch-based measurement systems are built. The use of variable maps and the guidelines for constructing measures in Chapter 4 are relevant for the rater accuracy issues explored in this chapter.

This chapter offers an illustration of how to construct a direct measure of rater accuracy that conceptualizes accuracy as a latent variable. Since accuracy is viewed as a latent variable and the rater is the object of measurement, the guidelines for constructing measures described in Chapter 4 can be used.

The sections covered in this chapter are:

- What is rater accuracy?
- Defining rater accuracy as a latent variable
- Indices of rating accuracy
- Illustrative data analyses
- Relationship between rater error and accuracy
- Summary and discussion

What is Rater Accuracy?

The literature on evaluating the quality of ratings is voluminous (Saal, Downey, & Lahey, 1980). In their extensive review of criteria used for evaluating ratings, Murphy and Cleveland (1995) identified three classes of rating quality indices: psychometric indices (e.g., reliability and inter-rater agreement), rater error indices (e.g., severity and halo error), and rating accuracy (e.g., elevation accuracy and halo accuracy). A key idea underlying the research on rating quality is that rater-mediated assessments define a process that requires the elicitation and analysis of expert judgments. The focus of rating-quality indices is on these rater judgments that become observable through a set of cues that define the lens used to define the judgmental processes of the raters. Brunswick's Lens model provides a useful way to begin to conceptualize these judgmental processes. The Facets Model, based on Rasch measurement theory, can be used to define assessment guidelines used to evaluate rating quality. The basic problem is to answer the following question: How can we evaluate the quality of ratings (judgments) obtained from a set of expert and trained raters within the context of various types of performance assessments?

Standard indices used for evaluating ratings have been dominated by inter-rater agreement indices. Rater agreement is the most commonly used index reported to support the inference that ratings are of high quality. Rater agreement indices view rater variation as a random and unsystematic bias in ratings. The next set of indices that have received a great deal of attention are called rater errors and biases, such as rater severity, halo effects, and response sets. These indices represent systematic biases that may perturb our rater-mediated assessment system, and the quality of the ratings.

The limitations of rater agreement indices have been identified in the literature. For example, Murphy and Cleveland (1995), state:

> Our overall conclusion is that rater error measures should be abandoned. They are based on arbitrary and often implausible assumptions, and there are too many nonequivalent definitions of each one. (p. 27)

Murphy and Cleveland (1995) suggest that rater agreement and rater error indices be replaced with more direct measures of rating accuracy. Some of the problems with indirect and traditional measures of rating quality can be addressed with Rasch-based indices for evaluating systematic errors and biases (Engelhard, 1994). These indirect measures of rating accuracy based on the Rasch model were described in Chapters 9 and 10 of this book.

A third category of rating quality indices can be defined in terms of rater accuracy. Accuracy can be defined as the comparison between unknown processes and a defined standard process in order to adjust the unknown process until it matches the standard. This is the essence of quality control processes (Shewhart, 1939). Indices of rating accuracy explore the discrepancies, differences and distances that result from the comparisons between observed and benchmark ratings. The benchmark ratings are defined as the standard or "true" ratings that would be assigned by an expert rater using the cues and processes defined by the rater-mediated assessment. Benchmark ratings can be defined in a variety of ways. One common approach is to combine or average ratings across a group of expert raters, and then to designate these ratings as the benchmark ("true") ratings. These benchmark ratings can be systematically used to directly evaluate the accuracy of observed ratings by embedding them within an operational assessment system. For example, the table below shows the ratings that three raters (Raters A, B, and C) rating two essays (Essays 1 and 2) using a 3-category rating scale assigned

	Observed rating		Benchmark Rating		Accuracy Rating		Accuracy Sum
Raters	*Essay 1*	*Essay 2*	*Essay 1*	*Essay 2*	*Essay 1*	*Essay 2*	
A	3	3	3	3	1	1	2
B	2	3	2	1	1	0	1
C	3	2	3	3	1	0	1
			Accuracy Sum:		3	1	4

The second and third columns contain those raters' observed ratings, while the fourth and fifth columns contain the mean benchmark ratings assigned by a panel of experts. The six and seventh columns contain the accuracy scores. These accuracy ratings are defined as follows: if the absolute value of the difference between the observed rating and the benchmark rating is 0, then the accuracy rating is 1; otherwise the accuracy rating 0. Accuracy ratings of one (A = 1) indicate perfect agreement, while accuracy scores of zero (A = 0) indicate discrepancies of 1 or greater between the observed and benchmark ratings. This hypothetical example indicates that this set of raters is more accurate when assigning ratings to Essay 1 than when assigning ratings to Essay 2. It also indicates that Rater A is more accurate than Raters B and C (last column). The overall accuracy of the ratings is 66.7% (4/6).

There are a variety of accuracy indices of rating quality that have been proposed in the literature (Jones, 2007). One straight forward index is the percent exact agreement between observed and benchmark ratings as shown in the example above. As is generally the case with rater agreement, it is also possible to calculate correlation coefficients between the observed and benchmark ratings. Another popular index is the D^2 index, and this accuracy index is defined as the mean square difference between the observed and benchmark ratings. D^2 is equivalent to percent exact agreement when the accuracy ratings are dichotomous (0 = inaccurate, 1 = accurate). Cronbach (1955) provided an early and influential discussion of accuracy ratings. He proposed the use of accuracy component scores that mimic the use of Generalizability Theory to identify various components of variance in observed ratings. Specifically, he identified the following accuracy components: elevation, differential elevation, stereotype accuracy, and differential accuracy. Sulsky and Balzer (1988) discuss other indices of rater accuracy and offer a thoughtful consideration of conceptual and computational issues related to an array of traditional indices and to rating accuracy.

As in other areas of measurement, advances in model-based measurement (Embretson, 1996) provide a useful framework for integrating these diverse indices into a family of indices for evaluating the psychometric quality of the measures. Engelhard (1996) proposed the use of Rasch-based indices of rating accuracy that address some of the limitations of the traditional indices, and this approach to rater accuracy is presented in the next section.

Defining Rater Accuracy as a Latent Variable

Four building blocks for constructing measures were described in Chapter 4. The four building blocks are the (a) latent variable, (b) observational design, (c) scoring rules, and (d) Rasch measurement model. The hypothesized variable map for the accuracy measure given in Figure 11.1. These building blocks are based on the approach proposed by Wilson (2005).

Logit Scale	Rater Accuracy	Benchmark Performance	Domain Accuracy	Rating Scale Structure
	[High accuracy]	*[Hard to be accurate]*	*[Hard to be accurate]*	*[High ratings]*
5.00	High values on the accuracy variable			
4.00				*4=very accurate*
3.00				
2.00				*3=accurate*
1.00				
.00	Midrange values on the accuracy variable	*[Moderately difficult to be accurate]*	*[Moderately difficult to be accurate]*	
-1.00				*2=minimal accuracy*
-2.00				
-3.00	Low values on the accuracy variable			
-4.00				*1=inadequate accuracy*
-5.00				
	[Low accuracy]	*[Easy to be accurate]*	*[Easy to be accurate]*	*[Low accuracy ratings]*

Figure 11.1 Hypothesized Variable Map for Measuring Rater Accuracy.

In this chapter, the underlying latent variable is rater accuracy, and the goal to objectively evaluate the correspondence between observed ratings and benchmark ratings (true ratings). The specific content area is communicative competence in writing. The observational design consists of the selection of a set of benchmark performances defined as written essays. These benchmark essays can be selected to represent a range of levels of proficiency in writing, and also to represent a range of different types of writing performances that may differ in terms of length and other essay characteristics. Once these benchmark essays are selected, then a panel of expert raters assigns ratings using a four-category rating scale (1 = low to 4 = high). The mean of the experts' ratings is defined as the "true rating" for a given essay. The scoring rule used to define accuracy ratings is as follows:

$$A_{ni} = \max\{|R_{ni} - B_i|\} - |R_{ni} - B_i| \qquad [1]$$

where R_{ni} is the observed rating from rater n on benchmark essay i, and B_i is the true rating on benchmark essay i. Although these accuracy ratings can vary from 0 to 3, previous research has suggested that dichotomous ratings (0 = inaccurate and 1 = accurate) provide useful accuracy ratings for illustrating the major points of this chapter. For example, a simple two-facet (raters and benchmark essays) dichotomous Rasch model can be used:

$$\ln\left[\frac{P_{ni1}}{P_{ni0}}\right] = \beta_n - \delta_i \qquad [2]$$

where P_{ni1} is the probability of rater n assigning an accurate rating (x = 1) on benchmark essay i, P_{ni0} is the probability of rater n assigning an inaccurate rating (x = 0) on benchmark essay i, β_n is the accuracy of rater n, and δ_i is the difficulty of assigning an accurate rating on benchmark essay i. The four building blocks for creating an accuracy scale are summarized in Table 11.1.

Engelhard (1996) proposed a Many Facet model for modeling accuracy ratings obtained from multiple raters on several domains (analytic scoring) with a four-category rating scale:

$$\text{Ln}\left[P_{nmik} / P_{nmik\text{-}1}\right] = \beta_n - \delta_m - \lambda_i - \tau_k \qquad [3]$$

where
P_{nmik} = probability of rater n assigning an accurate rating to benchmark essay m for domain i,
$P_{nmik\text{-}1}$ = probability of rater n assigning an inaccurate rating to benchmark essay m for domain i,
β_n = accuracy of rater n,
δ_m = difficulty of assigning an accurate rating to benchmark essay m,
λ_j = difficulty of assigning an accurate rating for domain i, and
τ_k = difficulty of accuracy-rating category k relative to category k–1.

Table 11.1   Four Building Blocks for Creating Variable Map for Rater Aaccuracy within the Context of Writing Assessment

Building Blocks	Questions	Answers	Rater-Accuracy Scale
Latent variable	What is the latent variable being measured?	Accuracy of raters in writing assessment	The purpose of the rater-accuracy scale is to objectively evaluate rater accuracy as the correspondence between observed ratings and benchmark ratings ("true ratings").
Observational design	What is the plan for collecting structured responses or observations from persons?	A set of benchmark performances are selected to represent a range of essays written in response to a writing prompt..	Raters read and score the essays using an analytic scale with four domains and four categories.
Scoring rules	How are responses or observations categorized to represent person levels on the latent variable?	The accuracy ratings are scored $x = 0$ (inaccurate) , $x = 1$ (accurate)	Operational raters are scored dichotomously based on whether their ratings match the benchmark ratings assigned by an expert panel.
Measurement model	How are person and item responses or observations mapped onto the latent variable?	Rasch model	Dichotomous Rasch model

Figure 11.2 provides the lens model for writing assessment that is represented by Equation 3. The idea behind the lens model is that rater accuracy is a latent variable that is made observable through a set of benchmark performances and through the particular domains that are selected.

Indices of Rating Accuracy

There are six aspects of accuracy: (a) rater accuracy, (b) halo accuracy (domain accuracy/true halo), (c) response-set accuracy, (d) score-range accuracy, (e) accuracy interaction effects, and (f) differential accuracy functioning. Table 11.2 summarizes the six aspects of accuracy by level of analysis and the question that each index helps to answer. This table is similar in structure to Table 10.2 in Chapter 10.

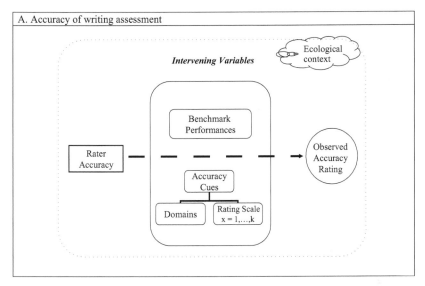

Figure 11.2 Lens Models for Rater Accuracy in Writing Assessment (Observed accuracy ratings).

There are a variety of statistical indices and graphical displays that can be used to evaluate rating accuracy based on the Many Facet Model. The three-facet model shown in Equation 3 (Raters, Benchmark Essays and Domains) is used to explore a set of accuracy-related research questions that are shown in Table 11.3.

Illustrative Data Analyses

This section continues the example from the previous chapter using writing data from Gyagenda and Engelhard (2010). The ratings from Rater 1 were actually obtained from a validity committee. The accuracy ratings in this section were computed using Equation 1, and then dichotomized to represent inaccurate (A = 0) and accurate (A = 1) ratings. The Many Facet model was fit to these data. Table 11.4 gives the overall summary statistics for the rater, domain and person facets of the model.

There are several things to note in this summary table. First of all, the rater facet is the object of measurement and it is not centered (M = .81, SD = .31). The convention in the Many Facet model is to center all of the other facets except the one that represents the object of measurement. This provides a stable frame of reference for interpreting the locations of raters, domains, and persons on the variable map. The summary fit statistics (Infit and Outfit) in Table 11.4 are within the expected values indicating good model-data fit. In

Table 11.2   Description of Rater Accuracy by Level of Analysis and Underlying
Questions

Definitions	*Level of Analysis*	
	Individual Raters	*Group of Raters*
Rater Accuracy: The tendency on the part of raters to consistently provide higher or lower ratings than warranted based on known person benchmarks.	How accurate is each rater? Where is the rater located on the variable map for accuracy?	Are the differences in rater accuracy significant? can the raters be considered of equivalent accuracy?
Halo accuracy (domain accuracy/true halo): Rater fails to distinguish between conceptually distinct and independent domains on person benchmarks.	Is the rater distinguishing between conceptually distinct and independent domains?	Are the raters distinguishing among the domains?
Response set accuracy: Rater interprets and uses rating scale categories in an idiosyncratic fashion. Rater overuses middle categories of rating scale when not warranted by person performance.	Is the rater using the rating scale as intended?	Are the raters using the rating scales as intended?
Score Range Accuracy: More or less variation in accuracy ratings of person benchmarks. Raters do not differentiate between person benchmarks on the latent variable.	How well did each rater differentiate among the person benchmarks?	Did the assessment system lead to the identification of meaningful person differences?
Accuracy interaction effects: Facets in the measurement model are not interpreted additively.	Is the rater interpreting and using the facets accurately?	Are the facets invariant across raters?
Differential accuracy functioning (DAF): Accuracy ratings are a function of construct-irrelevant components.	Are the accuracy ratings of each rater invariant over construct-irrelevant components?	Are the raters invariant over construct-irrelevant components for the overall assessment system?

addition to the summary statistics, the results for the rater and domain facets
are summarized in Tables 11.5 and 11.6.

The reliability of rater separation is statistically significant (*Rel* = .96, P
< .05). This indicates that this set of raters vary significantly in their lev-
els of accuracy. The accuracy measures range from 1.65 logits for Rater 10
(82% accuracy) to .44 logits for Rater 19 (60%). Table 11.5 provides additional

Table 11.3 Statistical Indices and Graphical Displays of Rating Accuracy based on the Many Facet Model (Raters, Domains and Benchmarks)

Indices and Displays	Rater Facet	Domain Facet	Benchmark Facet
1. Variable map	Where are the raters located on accuracy scale?	Where are the domains located on the accuracy scale?	Where are the persons' performances located on the accuracy scale?
2. Calibration and location of elements within facet	What is the location of each rater on the accuracy scale (low to high accuracy)?	How accurate are the raters when assigning ratings in each domain?	What is the judged location on the accuracy scale for person performances?
3. Standard errors for each element	How precisely has each rater been calibrated on the accuracy scale?	How precisely is each domain calibrated on the accuracy scale?	How precisely has the accuracy of each person performance been calibrated?
4. Reliability of separation	How spread out are the rater accuracy measures? Do the raters vary in accuracy?	Does rater accuracy vary across the domains?	Are the raters accurately distinguishing among persons' performances?
5. Chi-square statistic	Are the differences among the rater accuracy measures statistically significant?	Are the differences among the domain accuracy measures statistically significant?	Are the differences among the person accuracy measures statistically significant?
6. Mean square error (OUTFIT/ INFIT)	How accurately has each rater interpreted the person performances and domains?	How accurately has each domain been interpreted and used by the raters?	How accurately has person performance been interpreted by the raters?
7. Standardized residuals	How different is each accuracy rating from its expected value?	How different is each accuracy rating from its expected value?	How different is each accuracy rating from its expected value?
8. Quality control charts, figures and tables (displays of residuals)	What individual accuracy ratings appear to be higher or lower than expected based on the model?	What individual accuracy ratings appear to be higher or lower than expected based on the model?	What individual accuracy ratings appear to be higher or lower than expected based on the model?

(continued)

Table 11.3   Continued

Indices and Displays	Rater Facet	Domain Facet	Benchmark Facet
9. Interaction effects	Are there significant interaction effects between rater accuracy and other facets?	Are there significant interaction effects between domain accuracy and other facets?	Are there significant interaction effects between person performance accuracy and other facets?
10. Differential facet functioning	Is rater accuracy invariant across subgroups?	Is domain accuracy invariant across subgroups?	Is person performance accuracy invariant across raters?

information about the model-data fit for these raters. The domains also vary in terms of how difficult it is for raters to assign accurate ratings (Table 11.6): the mechanics domains (Mechanics/conventions and mechanics/sentence formation) tend to be easier to rate accurately in comparison to the meaning domains (Meaning/style and meaning/organization). These results are shown graphically on the variable map in Figure 11.3. The variable map indicates

Table 11.4   Summary Statistics for Accuracy Ratings

	Rater	Student	Domain
Measure			
Mean	.81	.00	.00
SD	.31	.63	.05
N	20	365	4
Outfit			
Mean	1.00	1.00	1.0
SD	.01	.03	<.00
Infit			
Mean	1.00	1.00	1.00
SD	.03	.09	.01
Separation statistic			
Reliability of separation	.96	.83	.84
Chi-square	622.8*	1348.7*	18.6*
(df)	(19)	(364)	(3)

* $p < .05$

Table 11.5   Accuracy Measures for Raters

Raters	Accuracy Agreement (Percents)	Measure Logits	S.E.	Infit MS	Outfit MS
10	0.82	1.65	0.05	1.01	1.06
2	0.78	1.36	0.06	1.00	0.98
4	0.75	1.19	0.06	1.00	1.00
6	0.73	1.07	0.06	1.02	1.04
11	0.69	0.88	0.06	0.96	0.93
12	0.69	0.88	0.06	0.99	0.99
17	0.69	0.86	0.06	1.00	0.99
14	0.68	0.81	0.06	1.00	1.00
8	0.67	0.77	0.06	0.99	1.02
20	0.67	0.76	0.06	1.00	1.03
9	0.66	0.71	0.06	1.00	0.98
13	0.66	0.74	0.06	0.99	0.96
3	0.65	0.67	0.06	1.03	1.05
16	0.65	0.71	0.06	1.00	1.00
15	0.64	0.63	0.06	1.02	1.02
5	0.62	0.54	0.06	1.00	0.98
18	0.61	0.52	0.06	1.00	1.01
21	0.61	0.49	0.06	1.01	1.01
7	0.60	0.45	0.06	0.99	0.98
19	0.60	0.44	0.06	1.00	0.98

Table 11.6   Accuracy Measures for Domains

Domains	Accuracy Agreement (Proportions)	Measure	S.E.	Infit MS	Outfit MS
Meaning/style	0.67	0.06	0.03	1.00	1.02
Meaning/ organization	0.67	0.04	0.03	1.00	1.01
Mechanics/ conventions	0.69	-0.03	0.03	1.00	1.00
Mechanics/ sentence formation	0.69	-0.07	0.03	0.99	0.98

```
|-----+-------------+-----------+-------|
|Logit|+Raters      |-Benchmarks|-Domains|
|-----+-------------+-----------+-------|
|     |  10         |           |        |
|     |  2          |           |        |
|     |             |           |        |
|     |  4          |  .        |        |
|     |  6          |           |        |
|  1 +|             +  .        +        |
|     |  11 12 17   |  *.       |        |
|     |  8   14 20  |  **.      |        |
|     |  3  9 13 16 |  *.       |        |
|     |  15         |  **.      |        |
|     |  5  7 18 21 |  ****.    |        |
|     |  19         |  *****    |        |
|     |             |  ******   |        |
|     |             |  ******   |        |
|     |             |  *******. | 1      |
| *  0 *            *  ******.  * 2 3   *
|     |             |  ***.     | 4      |
|     |             |  *******  |        |
|     |             |  ***      |        |
|     |             |  **.      |        |
|     |             |  **       |        |
|     |             |  *.       |        |
|     |             |  .        |        |
|     |             |  *.       |        |
|     |             |  .        |        |
| -1 +|             +  .        +        |
|     |             |  *        |        |
|     |             |  .        |        |
|     |             |           |        | 4,Domains
|     |             |  **.      |        | 1=Meaning/style
|-----+-------------+-----------+-------| 2=Meaning/organization
|Logit|+Raters      | * = 5     |-Domains| 3=Mechanics/conventions
+------------------------------------+    4=Mechanics/sentence formation
```

Figure 11.3 Variable map for accuracy scale.

that, by and large, this set of raters tended to assign accurate ratings to these benchmark essays with the targeting of the raters being located well above the benchmark essays in terms of their levels of accuracy.

Relationship Between Rater Error and Accuracy

A number of researchers have examined the congruence between rater error and bias indices and accuracy indices (e.g., Murphy & Cleveland, 1995). The general consensus is that rater error and bias indices are not useful indirect measures of rater accuracy. Recent research by Wind and Engelhard (2011) found that in some cases indirect measures may provide useful information about rater accuracy. As evidence to support this position, the correlations between selected rating quality measures are shown in Table 11.7.

Two of the striking correlations are the ones between rater accuracy and the Infit/Outfit mean square statistics obtained from the rater error analyses.

Table 11.7   Correlations among Indices of Rater Errors and Rater Accuracy

| | Rater Errors | | | Rater Accuracy | | |
	Severity	Infit	Outfit	Accuracy	A_Infit	A_Outfit
Severity	1.000	-.305	-.257	-.227	-.215	-.225
Infit	-.305	1.000	.946*	-.526*	.214	.167
Outfit	-.257	.946*	1.000	-.534*	.302	.271
Accuracy	-.227	-.526*	-.534*	1.000	.045	.270
A_Infit	-.215	.214	.302	.045	1.000	.793*
A_Outfit	-.225	.167	.271	.270	.793*	1.000

*p < .05

The plots of the accuracy measures and the Outfit mean square statistics for these 20 raters are shown in the two panels of Figure 11.4.

These plots indicate the strong relationship between the rater accuracy measures and the traditional Outfit mean square statistics that would be obtained from a Rasch analysis of rating data. Panel A shows the relationship for all 20 raters (r = −.534), and the even stronger relationship that appears when Rater 10 is removed from the analysis (r = −.772).

Discussion and Summary

In exact usage, precision is distinguished from accuracy. The latter refers to closeness of an observation to the quality intended to be observed. Precision is a quality associated with a class of measurements and refers to the way in which repeated observations conform to themselves; and in a somewhat narrower sense refers to the dispersion of the observations, or some measure of it, whether or not the mean value around which the dispersion is measured approximates to the "true" value.

(Kendall & Buckland, 1957, p. 224)

Stallings and Gillmore (1971) called for a stronger alignment between the terms reliability and validity with precision and accuracy:

The terms accuracy and precision are consistently differentiated in the literature of engineering and the "hard" sciences. Precision shares a common core of meaning with reliability as used by behavioral scientists. Accuracy and validity have a similar semantic overlap. (p. 127)

This chapter has introduced direct measures of rater accuracy and compared them to indirect measures of accuracy. These model-based indices obtained through the use of Rasch measurement theory offer the opportunity to

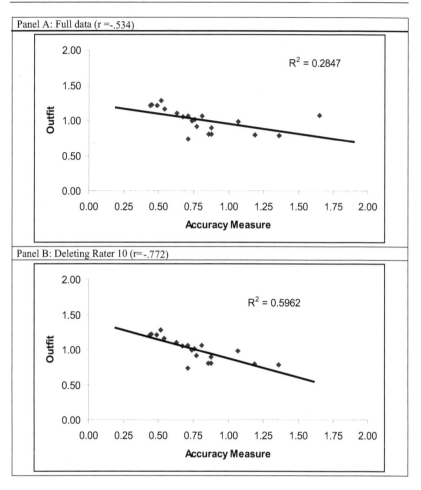

Figure 11.4 Plots of the relationships between accuracy measures and Outfit Statistics.

conceptualize accuracy as a latent variable to be measured in a manner similar to that used to measure other constructs in the social, behavioral and health sciences. The guiding principles of invariant measurement also undergird this perspective on rater accuracy. Engelhard (1996) and Engelhard, Davis, and Hansche (1999) have used the Many Facet model to examine rating accuracy.

Part V

Final Word

Chapter 12

Invariant Measurement
Discussion and Summary

I trust that the reader has been impressed by now with the fact that the theory of mental measurements is no display of mathematical pedantry or subtle juggling with figures, but on the contrary is simple common sense.

(Thorndike, 1904, p. 163)

The purpose of this book is to present an introduction to the concept of invariant measurement, and the use of the concept to explore measurement issues in the social, behavioral, and health sciences. Five requirements are introduced to organize our thinking about invariant measurement:

Person measurement:
1. The measurement of persons must be independent of the particular items that happen to be used for the measuring: Item-invariant measurement of persons.
2. A more able person must always have a better chance of success on an item than a less able person: non-crossing person response functions.

Item calibration:
3. The calibration of the items must be independent of the particular persons used for calibration: Person-invariant calibration of test items.
4. Any person must have a better chance of success on an easy item than on a more difficult item: non-crossing item response functions.

Variable map:
5. Items and person must be simultaneously located on a single underlying latent variable: variable map.

These five requirements can be used to guide and evaluate aspects of assessments in the social, behavioral, and health sciences. This book has concretely illustrated how Rasch measurement models can be used to meet these requirements. Other measurement models can also be used to explore aspects of invariant measurement (Millsap, 2011). In particular, exploratory measurement models that are based on nonparametric item response theories can be quite informative when the requirements of invariant measurement are not adequately approximated by real data (Sijtsma & Molenaar, 2002).

In the first four chapters, I provided an introduction to invariant measurement based on the Rasch model. The requirements of invariant measurement were described in Chapter 1 with the introduction of an illustrative data set designed to measure aspects of home environments. Chapters 2 and 3 provided descriptions of item-invariant person measurement and person-invariant item calibration based on a family of Rasch measurement models (Dichotomous Model, Partial Credit Model, Rating Scale Model, and Many Facet Model). A detailed description of how to construct measures based on Wilson's (2005) approach was included in Chapter 4.

Chapters 5 and 6 provided an historical and comparative perspective on the key ideas undergirding invariant measurement. In particular, Chapter 5 traced the development of two research traditions in measurement theory during the 20th century (the test-score tradition and the scaling tradition). Highlights of the quest for invariant measurement within the scaling tradition formed the core of the issues discussed in Chapter 6.

Rasch models can be viewed as ideal-type measurement theories that actualize the requirements of invariant measurement. In order to evaluate how well real data approximate these requirements, it is necessary to estimate the parameters of a Rasch model, and then to evaluate the goodness of fit between an ideal model and real data. Chapter 7 covered a variety of estimation methods that researchers and theorists have proposed for estimating the parameters in Rasch models, while Chapter 8 introduced a variety of ways to conceptualize model-data fit.

In Chapter 9, I introduced a conceptual framework that views raters and other aspects of rater-mediated assessments in terms of a lens model (Brunswik, 1952). This lens model is used to make visible the latent variable or construct that is being measured. The next two chapters suggested an array of indices that one can use to evaluate the quality of rater-mediated assessments using direct and indirect indicators of rater agreement, rater error and bias, and rater accuracy. One of the exciting areas for future research is the exploration of invariant measurement in assessment contexts that involve raters. In this final chapter, I briefly address topics related to perennial issues in assessment from the perspective of invariant measurement.

Perennial Issues in Assessment from the Perspective of Invariant Measurement

The principles of invariant measurement based on the Rasch model can provide useful perspectives and approaches for tackling a host of perennial and persistent methodological questions in the social, behavioral and health sciences. The issues discussed in this section are adapted from the work of Hattie, Jaeger, and Bond (1999). Figure 12.1 places invariant measurement in a

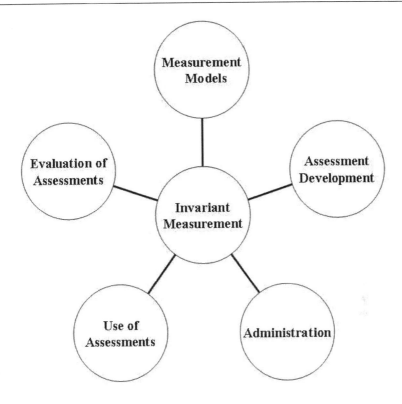

Figure 12.1   Perennial issues in measurement in the human sciences.

central role in addressing a set of five general measurement and assessment issues: conceptual models of measurement, assessment development, assessment administration, assessment use, and assessment evaluation (Hattie et al., 1999). This display is meant to portray the interactive nature of these aspects of assessment systems, as well as highlight the central role of the requirements of invariant measurement. The specific issues addressed here are:

- Measurement Models
- Assessment Development
- Administration of Assessments
- Use of Assessments
- Evaluation of Assessments

Measurement Models

One of the key themes of this book is that measurement models can function as paradigms and research traditions that guide the theory and practice of assessment in the human sciences. Theorists have developed a variety of measurement theories, but some theories are clearly better for evaluating the extent to which particular measurement contexts have met the requirements of invariant measurement. Chapter 5 presented a general framework for classifying measurement theories in terms of either a test score tradition or a scaling tradition. Much of the research work on classical test theory continues to be based on the "assumptions that errors of measurement are random and that the variances of such errors are the same for all examinees" (Hattie et al., 1999, p. 398). Classical test theory and other test-score based traditions cannot adequately conceptualize a separation of the characteristics of the persons from the characteristics of items and the test. Since item response theory has emerged as the dominant measurement theory in the 21st century (Embretson & Reise, 2000), it is important to fully embrace the underlying views of invariant measurement and model-based measurement within the scaling tradition.

One of the important outcomes of using model-based measurement, such as the Rasch model, is that an explicit theory-based foundation with the requirements of invariant measurement defined in detail can be constructed. If these requirements are met with real data, then it is possible to address a host of persistent measurement problems (Wright, 1977). The invariant measurement properties of the Rasch model have been known for some time, and successful applications continue to appear in the educational, social, behavioral and health sciences. For example, large-scale educational assessments with high-stakes in several states are built with Rasch models as a particular instantiations of invariant measurement. Variable maps provide simultaneous calibrations of both person locations on the latent variable and item difficulties on the same "rulers."

As was stressed in Chapter 4 in which I discussed Wilson's (2005) building blocks for researcher-constructed measures, the underlying measurement theory provides the guidance for assessment development, appropriate administration of the assessments, and reliable and valid use of the scores. Most importantly of all, measurement theories provide the criteria that one can use to evaluate the quality of the assessment system that has been constructed, and to support the inferences that are made on the basis of the assessment system. I strongly emphasize the choice of Rasch models as the underlying measurement models for building assessment systems because it yields the strongest opportunity to obtain invariant measurement. Other models, such as nonparametric IRT models, provide strategies for intermediate stages of assessment development along the way to achieving invariant measurement in the final scale.

In situations where invariant measurement is more difficult to achieve, other models, such as Generalizability Theory (Brennan, 2001; Cronbach, Gleser, Nanda, & Rajaratnam, 1972) with its focus on test scores, and Generalized Hierarchical Linear Models (Raudenbush & Bryk, 2002) can be used to help clarify aspects of the assessment process that may contribute to variant measurement.

Assessment Development

The use of Rasch measurement models provides guidance for all aspects of the assessment process including assessment development. Assessment development is a key building block that includes observational design and scoring rules (Wilson, 2005). Assessment development focuses on the design of items, tasks and other opportunities to elicit behavior from persons in order to draw inferences about each person's location on the latent variable of interest. In this section, the term "item" should be broadly conceived as any situation designed to obtain systematic information about person locations on a latent variable including various forms of selected and constructed response items or tasks. It is beyond the scope of this section to describe in detail all of the aspects of the item and test development processes, and Schmeiser and Welch (2006) should be consulted for a more comprehensive discussion of assessment development. The *Standards for Educational and Psychological Testing* (*Standards*; AERA, APA, & NCME, 1999) define four phases to consider in assessment development: (a) purpose of the assessment; (b) development of test specifications; (c) development, field testing, evaluation and selection of items, scoring guides and procedures for scoring; and (d) assessment and evaluation of the assessment for operational use.

From the perspective of invariant measurement, assessment development provides a proactive framework for creating and selecting assessment designs that offer objective and fair opportunities for persons to show where they are located on the variable map. In a sense, assessment development places more emphasis on the invariant measurement requirements related to item calibration with the goal of achieving person-invariant measurement: calibration of the items must be independent of the particular persons used for calibration, and persons must have a better chance of success on an easy item than on a more difficult item: non-crossing item response functions.

The principles of universal design (Johnstone, Altman, & Thurlow, 2006) hold great promise for guiding assessment development that supports invariant measurement. Universal design has its origins in architecture, and it provides principles that guide the creation of physical environments that persons with various disabilities can access. Ultimately, the goal is to create environments that everyone can access. Universal design principles are currently being extended into a variety of fields including the creation of assessment systems with a major focus on making assessments accessible to all, including persons with disabilities (Thurlow et al., 2008). Universal design offers a promising perspective for conceptualizing invariant measurement of persons with a variety of individual differences that can be mapped onto a common underlying latent variable.

Another important emergent perspective on assessment development is evidence-centered design (Huff, Steinberg, & Matts, 2010; Mislevy, Steinberg, Breyer, Almond, & Johnson, 2002). Evidence-centered assessment design (ECD; Mislevy et al., 2002) provides a framework for making sense of complex data. Evidence-centered assessment design explicitly considers how one can use assessment design to guide the collection of relevant evidence to support inferences based on test scores. Future research should fully explicate the connections between the principles of invariant measurement and the sound guidance for assessment development provided within the framework of evidence-centered design.

One important challenge in assessment development involves creating equivalent assessment forms composed of different subsets of items. For example, a number of states require graduation tests that carry very high stakes for students. In this situation, the same assessment form cannot be used from year to year because of test security concerns. It is essential that the scores on alternate forms of that assessment be comparable across years and equivalent over subsets of items nested within each form. The problem of equating assessments can be addressed in a variety of ways (Kolen & Brennan, 2004). Assessment developers may create item banks (Choppin, 1968) to aid in the creation of multiple invariant forms. These calibrated item banks can support the creation of computer-based and computer-adaptive assessments that represent a common latent variable that can yield equivalent scores. The goal is to create a set of items that are calibrated onto a common scale (variable map) that allows exchangeable estimates of person location based on different subsets of items.

Cognitive labs (Zucker, Sassman, & Case, 2004) have been used to gather evidence in support of the premise that the persons being assessed are interacting with the items and tasks in ways that are congruent with the theory of action that guided the assessment. The use of think-aloud protocols and other ways of analyzing verbal behaviors (Ericsson & Simon, 1999) can productively be used to examine and evaluate whether or not persons are responding in terms of cognitive operations as intended to assessment tasks. This research is particularly important within the context of assessing students who require various accommodations and modifications to access the assessments, such as students with disabilities and English language learners. Cognitive labs also can be used to ensure that innovative item formats are performing as intended to yield useful information about persons. In order to achieve item-invariant measurement of persons, it is essential to probe more deeply into the underlying cognitive processes that persons use as they interpret and respond to the assessment items and tasks.

Significant progress is being made on automated task development and test assembly (Drasgow, Luecht, & Bennett, 2006; Luecht, 1998). Automated assessment development offers another approach for creating invariant sets of assessment items and tasks that will yield exchangeable estimates of person location on the latent variable regardless of the particular items and tasks that are used to obtain these estimates.

Assessment development issues related to performance assessments can be productively viewed through the lens of rater-mediated assessments (Engelhard, 2002; Johnson, Penny, & Gordon, 2009). The essential issue is to seek tasks and prompts that create opportunities for persons to show what they know, what they can do, and what they need to learn next in a sequence of instruction. These behaviors and responses to the tasks should provide clear evidence that can be meaningfully interpreted by raters who are judging person responses. The assessment development process should include clear rubrics, and reflect an explicit concern with aiding raters to make judgments about person performances that are invariant across tasks.

Assessment development has evolved during the 20th century and continues to evolve into the 21st century. Researchers have carried out extensive research on item and assessment formats (Downing & Haladyna, 2006), although multiple-choice items continue to dominate assessment practices. Main guiding issues for assessment development from the perspective of invariant measurement are related to design of items, tasks, and prompts that provide useful information indicative of person locations on the latent variable or construct being measured. This information should not be overly dependent on the particular mode of assessment or particular person characteristics that may be construct irrelevant. Research questions regarding the invariance of person locations on the latent variable over varying formats is a very active area of research. This includes a consideration of assessment development issues that can be used to support invariant measurement within the context of computer-adaptive assessments. As pointed out by Schmeiser and Welch (2006), "we continue to strive for the right balance between art and the science of test development (p. 351). The principles of invariant measurement can contribute to further progress in assessment development.

Administration of Assessments

Issues concerning the administration of assessments place more relative emphasis on the invariant measurement requirements related to item-invariant measurement of persons: measurement of persons must be independent of the particular items that happen to be used for the measuring, and more able persons must always have a better chance of success on an item than less able persons.

Group-based administrations of tests composed of multiple-choice items have been used since World War I with the Army Alpha Tests. These large-scale administrations of tests have persisted into the 21st century. Group-based administrations of standardized assessments are sometimes viewed as inauthentic as compared to performance assessments, but their efficiency and apparent fairness (as defined by the principle that all students experience the same administration conditions) contribute to the persistence of group-based administrations of many standardized assessments.

Performance assessments may be somewhat less standardized and more authentic, but the issues of reliability and validity of the scores based on these assessments pose a host of measurement issues and problems. As pointed out in Chapters 9–11, the development of psychometrically sound rater-mediated assessment systems that support rater-invariant measurement is not a trivial activity.

Accommodations and modifications of the standardized testing for persons with disabilities and other special needs, such as persons assessed in a different language, can also be productively viewed through the lens of invariant measurement. In this case, the principle of invariant measurement focuses on the issue of how to appropriately adapt or modify the assessment protocols to yield accurate estimates of the location of these persons in terms of what they know and are able to do. In particular, invariant measurement can be used as a framework for examining differential item functioning and differential person functioning (Engelhard, 2009a).

Computer adaptive testing (CAT) offers an attractive alternative to traditional paper-and-pencil assessments. The promise of CAT is for faster estimation of scores with the use of fewer and targeted items appropriately administered to each person. Some challenges still remain, such as the need to develop psychometrically sound large calibrated item banks that can assure invariant measurement for all persons responding to items administered in a CAT-based assessment system.

Use of Assessments

Invariant measurement stresses person-invariant item calibration and item-invariant measurement of persons. When these requirements are approximated, then an important step has been taken in ensuring that the scores have conceptually defensible meaning that can undergird the appropriate interpretation and use of test scores. Invariance across person characteristics (no differential item functioning), invariance across item characteristics (no differential person functioning), and invariant interpretations across different contexts are fundamental for invariant measurement in the human sciences.

Assessments are developed to be used to inform a variety of decisions. The purpose of an assessment is defined by the intended use of scores, and the purpose is an essential consideration in all aspects of the assessment process. Unfortunately, test-score users are not always aware of how closely linked the intended use of assessments is to every phase of the process, from the specification of content, through choices regarding measurement models, to criteria used to examine the psychometric quality of the assessment. It is essential to re-evaluate an assessment system when test scores are used for purposes that the assessment developers did not intend.

Setting standards for test performances has emerged as an essential aspect of the use of assessment. Performance standards defined by cut scores that categorize persons on the underlying latent variable are used to make numerous decisions in the human sciences. Cizek and Bunch (2007) describe a variety of methods for setting cut scores. The principles of invariant measurement have begun to be applied for evaluating the quality of judgments obtained from panelists on standard-setting committees (Engelhard, 2009b).

Evaluation of Assessments

In a sense, this whole book has been about the evaluation of assessments from the perspective of invariant measurement. The internal structure of the assessment can be evaluated based on model-data fit considerations guided by the Rasch measurement model. Other important aspects of the evaluation of assessments can be related to the external structure of the assessments in terms of recommended and appropriate uses of scores within different contexts. The *Standards* provide good advice for selecting appropriate methods to gather reliability evidence, as well as validity evidence, to support the inferences made from test scores.

Historically, the two concepts of reliability and validity have dominated the discussions of the psychometric quality of the measures developed in the human sciences. Reliability estimates provide information regarding the consistency of scores. In essence, reliability can be viewed as the invariance of person ordering over various potential sources of error variance, such as the time of administration and different subsets of items. From the perspective of the test-score tradition discussed in Chapter 5, reliability coefficients provide information regarding sources of error variance in observed test scores. Evidence of test-score consistency is sample-dependent, and it is usually presented in terms of a variety of different reliability coefficients including test-retest reliability, equivalent-forms reliability, and various internal consistency estimates of reliability (e.g., Kuder-Richardson Formulas 20 and 21, Cronbach's coefficient alpha, etc.). Linn, Gronlund, and Miller (2008) should be consulted for descriptions of classical definitions and uses of a variety of reliability coefficients.

Invariant measurement, as reflected in Rasch measurement theory, provides a slightly different perspective on test-score reliability and standard errors of measurement. Standard errors of measurement are minimized (and reliability coefficients maximized) when the items are targeted to the person locations on the latent variable. In Rasch measurement theory, the reliability of the person separation index is similar to coefficient alpha. The reliability of separation is the ratio of true score variance to total observed score variance. Wright and Masters (1982) describe in detail how the concept of "reliability" is interpreted within the context of Rasch measurement theory.

Validity evidence can also be used to evaluate the psychometric quality of assessment systems. One of the major conceptual developments in measurement during the late 20th century was the recognition that validity can only be meaningfully approached from a consideration of the intended and appropriate use of test scores to make decisions and inferences within a particular context (Messick, 1989). The contexts of uses for test scores vary considerably in the social, behavioral and health sciences. In educational settings, test scores are used to make decisions about students (high graduation), teachers (evaluation of teacher performance), and schools (quality of the education provided). The important point from a validity perspective is that each of the intended uses must be supported with relevant and appropriate types of evidence. The Standards (AERA, APA, & NCME, 1999) recommend collecting evidence to build a sound and convincing validity argument to support the use of test scores for making particular decisions. The Standards also stress the importance of gathering validity evidence for determining the psychometric quality of an assessment. This includes the interpretation and use of scores within the context of theory, research and practice. Wilson (2005) should be consulted for a more detailed treatment of how scaling theory addresses the concepts of reliability and validity.

Final Word

This book has covered a wide range of topics related to invariant measurement in general, and the use of the Rasch measurement model in particular to explore these issues. Future developments in measurement theory are likely to focus on clarifying fixed and random effects models, and the connections of these models to the requirements and guiding principles of invariant measurement (de Boeck & Wilson, 2004). I also envision an expanded role for non-parametric item response models in increasing our understanding of how invariant measurement can be employed productively at various stages of measurement and research processes in the social, behavioral and health sciences. Although the development of new measurement models is important, research is needed on the consolidation, interpretation, and use of current models. In particular, the translations of measurement theories into sound measurement practices are expected to play a key role in contributing to progress in the human sciences.

My overarching goal in this book has been to whet the appetite of the reader to delve more deeply into the issues related to invariant measurement. In particular, an overall commitment by scholars to the improvement of measurement based on the principles of invariant measurement holds great promise for progress in research, theory, and practice within the human sciences.

Glossary

Ability   The general term used to describe the level of performance of a person on a latent variable as measured by an assessment.

Bloom's Taxonomy   A classification of learning objectives developed by Bloom et al. (1956) based on six cognitive levels: knowledge, comprehension, application, analysis, synthesis, and evaluation.

Birnbaum Models (2PL, 3PL)   Measurement models proposed by Birnbaum (1968) using the logistic item response function that include a two parameter logistic (2PL) model with item and slope parameters, as well as a three parameter logistic (3PL) model that adds a guessing parameter.

Calibration   The process of estimating the location of items on the variable map.

Category Response Function   A function that represents the relationship between the probability of selecting a response category and the underlying latent variable.

Construct (Latent variable)   Underlying variable that is represented by the variable map.

Deterministic Models   Measurement models to reflect ideal types or theories regarding person responses to test items that are not probabilistic (stochastic).

Dichotomous Data   These are response outcomes that are divided into two non-overlapping categories (e.g., not present/present, yes/no, and wrong/right).

Dichotomous Model   Rasch measurement model used to analyze dichotomous data.

Differential Item Functioning (DIF)   The examination of the conditional probabilities of success on an item between subgroups that have comparable locations on the latent variable.

Differential person functioning   Method used for examining unexpected differences between the observed and expected performance of persons on a set of items.

Double Monotonicity   A term used to describe non-crossing item and person response functions.

Facets   A computer program designed to apply Rasch measurement theory to person-item response data (http://winsteps.com/facets.htm).

Four Building Blocks   A set of guidelines proposed by Wilson (2005) to guide the construction of measures based on a latent variable, observational design, scoring rule, and measurement model.

Generalizability Theory   An approach to measurement proposed by Cronbach et al. (1972) that extends classical test theory to include multiple sources of measurement error.

Goodness-of-fit   A judgment of how well a data set fits a measurement model.

Guttman Scaling   A technique for examining whether or not a set of items administered to a group of persons is unidimensional as proposed by Guttman.

Ideal-Type Model   A measurement model that specifies the requirements to be met in order to realize desirable measurement properties, such as invariant measurement.

Invariant Measurement   A philosophical approach to measurement that supports item-invariant measurement of persons and person-invariant calibration of items that can be simultaneously represented by a variable map.

Items   A general set of stimuli or tasks intended to provide a structural framework for obtaining person responses that are used to infer person locations on a latent variable.

Item Characteristic Curve   This is another name for item response functions as used in this book.

Item difficulty   This is the location of the item on the latent variable in log-odds units (logits).

Item-Invariant Person Measurement   The measurement of persons should be independent of the particular items used to assign a location of a person on a latent variable.

Item Response Function (IRF)   A function that represents the relationship between person locations on the latent variable and probability of a positive response on an item.

Latent variable   The underlying construct that is being measured or represented by variable map.

Logits (Logit Scale)   Underlying scale units that are obtained by a logistic transformation of item response probabilities.

Many Facet Model   A Rasch measurement model that can be used to model data that has multiple facets (Linacre, 1989).

Measurement   The systematic process of locating both persons and items on a variable map that represents a latent variable (construct).

Model-Data Fit   A judgment of the degree to which the data under investigation meets the requirements of a measurement model.

Monotonicity   The direction of the cumulative probability of response functions that can be used to examine the hypotheses related to invariant measurement.

Normits   These are units in the field of biometrics based on a transformation of proportions based on the normal curve that are similar in form to logits used in Rasch measurement models.

Nonparametric Model   A model that does not limit the form of the underlying operating characteristic function to a particular type.

Objective Measurement   The phrase used by Benjamin Wright to describe Rasch's concept of specific objectivity. Essentially, equivalent to the concept of invariant measurement as described in the book.

Observational Design   A set of rules for systematically generating item and stimulus situations to obtain responses from persons.

Operating characteristic function (OCF)   The OCF represents the general form of the item or person response functions that are used to stochastically model measurement data.

Operational Definition   A detailed definition of a latent variable represented in invariant measurement by the variable map.

Parameter Separation   A property of Rasch measurement models that allows the conditional separation of item and person locations on the latent variable.

Parametric Models   These models specify a priori the structure of the underlying operating characteristic functions.

Partial Credit Model   A unidimensional Rasch model for ratings in two or more ordered categories.

Perfect Scale   This is another name for a Guttman Scale.

Persons   This is the object of measurement, and it is synonymous with other terms, such as subjects, participants, examinees, respondents, and individuals.

Person Measures   The location of persons on a latent variable in log-odd units (logits).

Person-Invariant Item Calibration   The requirement that the location of items should be independent of the particular persons used to assign a location of an item on a latent variable.

Person Response Function   The function that represents the relationship between response probabilities and a set of items for a person.

Polytomous   These are response outcomes that are divided into more than two non-overlapping categories (e.g., low/medium/high; strongly disagree/ disagree/agree/strongly agree).

Population of Objects   The target group of persons that the scale is designed to measure.

Probabilistic Models   These are statistical models that estimate the probability of an event occurring based on a set of known data

Rater-Mediated Assessment   Any assessment or test that consists of constructed-responses that require a rater, reader, judge or examiner to interpret the performance and to assign a judgment rating.

Rasch Measurement Models   A family of measurement models that provide an opportunity to meet the five requirements of invariant measurement including the following models: Dichotomous Model, Partial-Credit Model, Rating-Scale Model, and Many-Facet Model.

Rating Scale   Structure of the format used to collect numerical ratings (e.g., Likert scale).

Rating Scale Model   A unidimensional Rasch model that can be used to analyze ratings in two or more ordered categories.

Researcher-Constructed Measures   An approach for constructing measures based on the four building blocks proposed by Mark Wilson.

Research Traditions   A concept developed by Laudan (1977) to describe the underlying paradigms that guide the practice of science in a variety of disciplines.

Response Format   The method used to collect responses from persons (e.g., multiple-choice and constructed response items).

Scaling Tradition   A set of measurement theories, such as Rasch measurement theory and item response theory that focuses on item and person responses with the goal of achieving invariant measurement.

Scalogram Analysis   This is another name for Guttman Scaling.

Scoring Rubric   The guidelines used to define and score responses to constructed-response items, such as essays.

Scoring Rules   These are detailed description of how to map categories of observations into scores that are used in a measurement model.

Specific Objectivity   Rasch (1960/1980) used this term to describe his version of invariant measurement. The concept is similar to objective measurement as used by Wright (1968).

Test-Score Tradition   A set of measurement theories, such as classical test theory and generalizability theory that focuses on test scores, and the sources of error variance that may affect the interpretation and use of test scores.

Unidimensional   A term used to describe a meaningful mapping of persons and items onto a single construct represented by a variable map.

Variable map   A visual representation of the construct being measured. Variable maps have also been called construct maps, item maps, curriculum maps, and Wright maps.

Notation

Items

δ_i	Location of item i on the latent variable
L	Number of items
$\hat{\delta}$	Estimate of item difficulty in logits
$\bar{\delta}$	Mean item difficulties in logits
$\hat{\sigma}_\delta^2$	Variance of item difficulties in logits

Persons

θ_n	Location of person n on the latent variable
N	Number of persons
x_{ni}	Observed response from person n to item i
$\hat{\theta}$	Estimate of person location in logits
$\bar{\theta}$	Mean location of persons in logits
$\hat{\sigma}_\theta^2$	Variance of person locations in logits

Functions

$\Psi(x) = \dfrac{\exp(x)}{1+\exp(x)}$	Cumulative distribution function (logistic distribution)
$\Psi(x_{ni}) = P_{ni} = \Psi(\theta_n - \delta_i)$	Probability of person n succeeding on item i
$P_{Ai} = \Psi(\theta_A - \delta_i)$	Person Response Function for Person A
$P_{n1} = \Psi(\theta_n - \delta_1)$	Item Response Function for Item 1
$\phi_{ni1} = \dfrac{\exp(\theta_n - \delta_{i1})}{1+\exp(\theta_n - \delta_{i1})}$	Operating characteristic function
$\pi_{ni1} = \dfrac{\exp(\theta_n - \delta_{i1})}{1+\exp(\theta_n - \delta_{i1})}$	Category characteristic function

Note. Exceptions to this notation are noted as needed within the text of the book.

References

Adams, R. J., & Wilson, M. R. (1996). A random coefficients multinomial logit: A generalized approach to fitting Rasch models. In G. Engelhard and M. Wilson (Eds.), *Objective measurement III: Theory into practice* (pp. 143–166). Norwood, NJ: Ablex.

Adams, R. J., Wilson, M. R., & Wang, W. C. (1997). The multidimensional random coefficients multinomial logit. *Applied Psychology Measurement, 21*, 1–24.

Andersen, E. B. (1980). *Discrete statistical models with social science applications.* Amsterdam: North-Holland Publishing.

Adams, R. J., & Wu, M. L. (Eds.). (2002). *PISA 2000 Technical Report.* Paris: OECD Publications.

Agresti, A. (1990). *Categorical data analysis.* New York: Wiley.

American Educational Research Association, American Psychological Association, and National Council on Measurement in Education (1999). *Standards for educational and psychological testing.* Washington, DC: AERA.

Anderson, E. B. (1973). Conditional inference for multiple-choice questionnaires. *British Journal of Mathematical and Statistical Psychology, 26*, 31–44.

Anderson, L. W., & Sosniak, L. A. (Eds.). (1994). *Bloom's taxonomy: A forty-year retrospective.* Chicago: The University of Chicago Press.

Andrich, D. A. (1978a). Application of a psychometric model to ordered categories which are scored with successive integers. *Applied Psychological Measurement, 2*, 581–594.

Andrich, D. A. (1978b). A rating formulation for ordered response categories. *Psychometrika, 43*, 561–573.

Andrich, D. (1982). An index of person separation in latent trait theory, the traditional KR.20 indices and the Guttman scale response pattern. *Education Research and Perspectives*, 9, 95–104.

Andrich, D. A. (1985). An elaboration of Guttman scaling with Rasch models for measurement. In N. B. Tuma (Ed.), *Sociological methodology* (pp. 33–80). San Francisco: Jossey-Bass.

Andrich, D. A. (1988). *Rasch models for measurement.* Newbury Park, CA: Sage.

Andrich, D. (1989). Distinctions between assumptions and requirements in measurement in the social sciences. In J. A. Keats, R. Taft, R. A. Heasth, & S. H. Lovibond (Eds.), *Mathematical and Theoretical Systems* (pp. 7–16). North Holland: Elsevier Science.

Andrich, D. A., de Jong, J. H. A. L., & Sheridan, B. E. (1997). Diagnostic opportunities with the Rasch model for ordered response categories. In J. Rost & R. Langeheine (Eds.), *Applications of latent trait and latent class models in the social sciences* (pp. 59–70). Munster, Germany: Waxman Verlag Gmbh.

Andrich, D., Lyne, A., Sheridan, B., & Luo (2000). *RUMM2010 Computer Program.* Perth, Australia: Rumm Laboratory.

Ashton, W. D. (1972). *The logit transformation with special reference to its uses in bioassay.* New York: Hafner.

Baker, F. B., & Kim, S. (2004). *Item response theory: Parameter estimation techniques. Second edition, Revised and expanded.* New York: Marcel Dekker.

Barndorf-Nielsen, O. (1978). *Information and exponential families in statistical theory.* New York: Wiley.

Biggs, J. B., & Collis, K. F. (1982). *Evaluating the quality of learning: The SOLO taxonomy.* New York: Academic Press.

Birnbaum, A. (1957). *Efficient design and use of tests of a mental ability for various decision making problems.* Series Report No. 58-16, Project No. 7755-23. Randolph Air Force Base, Texas: USAF Scholl of Aviation Medicine.

Birnbaum, A. (1958a). *On the estimation of mental ability.* Series Report No. 15, Project No. 7755-23. Randolph Air Force Base, Texas: USAF Scholl of Aviation Medicine.

Birnbaum, A (1958b). *Further considerations of efficiency in tests of a mental ability.* Series Report No. 58-17, Project No. 7755-23. Randolph Air Force Base, Texas: USAF School of Aviation Medicine.

Birnbaum, A. (1968). Some latent trait models and their use in inferring an examinee's ability, Part 5. In F. M. Lord & M. R. Novick (Eds.), *Statistical theories of mental test scores* (pp. 395–479). Reading, MA: Addison-Wesley.

Bloom, B. S. (1970). Toward a theory of testing which includes measurement-evaluation-assessment (pp. 25–50). In M. C. Wittrock & D. Wiley (Eds.). *Evaluation of instruction: Issues and practices.* New York: Holt, Rhinehart and Winston.

Bloom, B .S., Englehart, M. D., Furst, E. J., Hill, W. H., & Krathwohl, D. R. (1956). *Taxonomy of educational objectives, the classification of educational goals: Handbook I: The cognitive domain.* New York: McKay.

Bock, R. D. (1997). A brief history of item theory response. *Educational Measurement: Issues and Practice, 16*(4), 21–33.

Bock, R. D., & Aitkin, M. (1981). Marginal maximum likelihood estimation of item parameters: Application of an EM algorithm. *Psychometrika, 46,* 443–459.

Bock, R. D., Gibbons, R., & Muraki, E. (1988). Full-information item factor analysis. *Applied Psychological Measurement, 12*(3), 261–280.

Bock, R. D., & Jones, L. V. (1968). *The measurement and prediction of judgment and choice.* San Francisco: Holden-Day.

Bock, R. D., & Moustaki, I. (2007). Item response theory in a general framework. In C. R. Rao & S. Sinharay (Eds.), *Psychometrics, Handbook of statistics* (Vol. 26, pp. 469–514). Amsterdam: Elsevier.

Boehm, A. E. (1985). Review of the Home Observation for Measurement of the Environment. In J. V. Mitchell, Jr. (Ed.), *9th Mental Measurements Yearbook* (pp. 663–665) Lincoln: University of Nebraska Press.

Bond, T. G., & Fox, C. M. (2007). *Applying the Rasch model: Fundamental measurement in the human sciences* (2nd ed.). Mahwah, NJ: Erlbaum.

Borg, I., & Shye, S. (1995). *Facet theory: Form and content.* Thousand Oaks, CA: Sage.

Brennan, R. L. (1997). A perspective on the history of generalizability theory. *Educational measurement: Issues and practice, 16*(4), 14–20.

Brennan, R. L. (2001). *Generalizability theory.* New York: Springer-Verlag.

Brigham, C. C. (1934). *The reading of the comprehensive examination in English: An analysis of the procedures followed during the five reading periods from 1929– 1933.* Princeton, NJ: Princeton University Press.

Brown, C. W., Bartelme, P., & Cox, G. M. (1933). The scoring of individual performance on tests scaled according to the theory of absolute scaling. *Journal of Educational Psychology, 24*(9), 654–662.

Brunswick, E. (1952). *The conceptual framework of psychology.* Chicago: University of Chicago Press.

Brunswik, E. (1956). *Perception and the representative design of psychological experiments.* (2nd ed.). Berkeley: University of California Press.

Caldwell, B. M., & Bradley, R. H. (1984). *Home observation for measurement of environment.* Little Rock: University of Arkansas Press.

Cattell, J. M. (1893). Mental measurement. *Philosophical Review, 2,* 316–332.

Choppin, B. (1968). Item bank using sample-free calibration. *Nature, 21* (August 24), 870–872.

Choppin, B. (1985). A fully conditional estimation procedure for Rasch model parameters. *Evaluation in Education, 9,* 29–42.

Choppin, B. (1987). The Rasch model for item analysis. In D. I. McArthur (Ed.), *Alternative approaches to the assessment of achievement* (pp. 99–127). Norwell, MA: Kluwer.

Cizek, G. J., & Bunch, M. B. (2007). *Standard setting: A guide to establishing and evaluating performance standards on tests.* Thousand Oaks, CA: Sage.

Cliff, N. (1983). Evaluating Guttman scales: Some old and new thoughts. In H. Wainer & S. Messick (Eds.), *Principles of modern psychological measurement: A festschrift for Frederic M. Lord* (pp. 283–301). Hillsdale, NJ: Erlbaum.

Cliff, N., & Keats, J. A. (2003). *Ordinal measurement in the behavioral sciences.* Mahwah, NJ: Erlbaum.

Clifford, G. J. (1984). *Edward L. Thorndike: The sane positivist.* Middletown, CT: Wesleyan University Press.

Cochran, W. G. (1952). The χ^2 test of goodness of fit. *Annals of Mathematical Statistics, 23,* 315–345.

Cohen, L. (1979). Approximate expressions for parameter estimates in the Rasch model. *British Journal of Mathematical and Statistical Psychology, 32,* 13–120.

Coser, L. A. (1977). *Masters of sociological thought: Ideas in historical and social context* (2nd ed.). Fort Worth, TX: Harcourt Brace Jovanovich.

Cressie, N., & Read, T. R. C. (1988). Cressie-Read statistic. In S. Kotz & N. L. Johnson (Eds.), *Encyclopedia of statistical sciences, supplementary volume* (pp. 37–39) New York: Wiley.

Crocker, L., & Algina, J. (1986). *Introduction to classical and modern test theory.* New York: Holt, Rinehart and Winston.

Cronbach, L. J. (1951). Coefficient alpha and the internal structure of tests. *Psychometrika, 16*, 297–334.

Cronbach, L. (1955). Processes affecting scores on "understanding of others" and "assumed similarity". *Psychological Bulletin, 52*, 177–193.

Cronbach, L. J. (1957). The two disciplines of scientific psychology. *American Psychologist, 12*, 671–684.

Cronbach, L. J. (1975). Beyond the two disciplines of scientific psychology. *American Psychologist*, 116–127.

Cronbach, L. J., Rajaranam, N., & Gleser, G. C. (1963). Theory of generalizability: A liberalization of reliability theory. *British Journal of Statistical Psychology, 16*, 137–163.

Cronbach, L. J., Gleser, G. C., Nanda, H., & Rajaratnam, N. (1972). *The dependability of behavioral measurements: Theory of generalizability for scores and profiles.* New York: Wiley.

Cuban, L. (1990). Four stories about national goals for American education. *Phi Delta Kappan*, (December), 265–271.

Cudeck, R., & MacCallum, R. C. (Eds.). (2007). *Factor analysis at 100: Historical developments and future directions.* Mahwah, NJ: L. Erlbaum.

de Boeck, P., & Wilson, M. (Eds.). (2004). *Explanatory item response models: A generalized nonlinear approach.* New York: Springer.

Downing, S. M., & Haladyna, T. M. (2006). *Handbook of test development.* Erlbaum.

Drasgow, F., Luecht, R. M., & Bennett, R. E. (2006). Technology and testing. In R.L. Brennan (Ed.), *Educational measurement, 4th edition* (pp. 471–515). Westport, CT: Praeger.

du Toit, M. (Ed.). (20003). *IRT from SSI: BILOG-MG, MULTILOG, PARSCALE, and TESTFACT.* Lincolnwood, IL: Scientific Software International.

DuBois, P. H. (1970). *A history of psychological testing.* Boston: Allyn and Bacon.

Duckor, B., Draney, K., & Wilson, M. (2009). Measuring measuring: Toward a theory of proficiency with the constructing measures framework. *Journal of Applied Measurement, 10*(3), 296–319.

Ebel, R. L. (1951). Estimation of the reliability of ratings. *Psychometrika, 16*, 407–424.

Edgeworth, F. Y. (1890). The element of chance in competitive examinations. *Journal of Royal Statistical Society, 53*, 460–475, 644–663.

Ellis, B. (1968). *Basic concepts in measurement.* Cambridge, UK: Cambridge University Press.

Embretson, S. E. (1996). The new rules of measurement. *Psychological Assessment, 8*(4), 341–349.

Embretson, S. E. (Ed.). (2010). *Measuring psychological constructs: Advances in model-based approaches.* Washington, DC: American Psychological Association.

Embretson, S. E., & Reise, S. P. (2000). *Item response theory for psychologists.* Mahwah, NJ: Erlbaum.

Enders, C. K. (2005). Maximum likelihood estimation. In B. S. Everitt & D. C. Howell (Eds.), *Encyclopedia of statistics in behavioral science, Volume 3* (pp. 1164–1170). Chicester, UK: Wiley.

Engelhard, G. (1984). Thorndike, Thurstone and Rasch: A comparison of their methods of scaling psychological and educational tests. *Applied Psychological Measurement, 8*, 21–38.

Engelhard, G. (1991). Thorndike, Thurstone and Rasch: A comparison of their approaches to item-invariant measurement. *Journal of Research and Development in Education,* 24(2), 45–60.

Engelhard, G. (1992). Historical views of invariance: Evidence from the measurement theories of Thorndike, Thurstone and Rasch. *Educational and Psychological Measurement,* 52(2) 275–292.

Engelhard, G. (1994a). Examining rater errors in the assessment of written composition with a many-faceted Rasch model. *Journal of Educational Measurement, 31*(2), 93–112.

Engelhard, G. (1994b). Historical views of the concept of invariance in measurement theory. In M. Wilson (Ed.), *Objective measurement: Theory into practice, volume 2* (pp. 73–99). Norwood, NJ: Ablex.

Engelhard, G. (1996). Evaluating rater accuracy in performance assessments. *Journal of Educational Measurement, 33*(1), 56–70.

Engelhard, G. (2002). Monitoring raters in performance assessments. In G. Tindal & T. Haladyna (Eds.), *Large-scale assessment programs for all students: Development, implementation, and analysis* (pp. 261–287). Mahwah, NJ: Erlbaum.

Engelhard, G. (2005a). Guttman scaling. In K. Kempf-Leonard (Ed.), *Encyclopedia of social measurement* (Vol. 2., pp. 167–174). San Diego, CA: Academic Press.

Engelhard, G. (2005b). Item Response Theory (IRT) models for rating scale data. *Encyclopedia of statistics in behavioral science (Vol. 2)* (pp. 995–1003). Hoboken, NJ: Wiley.

Engelhard, G. (2008a). Historical perspectives on invariant measurement: Guttman, Rasch, and Mokken [Special issue]. *Measurement: Interdisciplinary Research and Perspectives* (6), 1–35.

Engelhard, G. (2008b). Tuneable goodness-of-fit statistics. *Rasch Measurement Transactions, 22*(1), 1158–1159.

Engelhard, G. (2009a). Using IRT and model-data fit to conceptualize differential item and person functioning for students with disabilities. *Educational and Psychological Measurement, 69*(4), 585–602.

Engelhard, G. (2009b). Evaluating the judgments of standard-setting panelists using Rasch Measurement Theory. In E. V. Smith, Jr., & G. E. Stone (Eds.), *Criterion referenced testing: Practice analysis to score reporting using Rasch measurement models* (pp. 312–346). Maple Grove, MN: JAM Press.

Engelhard, G., Davis, M., & Hansche, L. (1999). Evaluating the accuracy of judgments obtained from item review committees. *Applied Measurement in Education, 12*(2), 199–210.

Engelhard, G., & Myford, C. M. (2003). *Monitoring faculty consultant performance in the Advanced Placement English Literature and Composition Program with a many-faceted Rasch model.* New York: College Entrance Examination Board.

Engelhard, G., & Osberg, D. W. (1983). Constructing a test network with a Rasch measurement model. *Applied Psychological Measurement, 7,* 283–294.

Ericsson, K. A., & Simon, H. A. (1999). *Protocol analysis: Verbal reports as data.* Cambridge, MA: Massachusetts Institute of Technology.

Fechner, G. T. (1860). *Elemente der psychophysik* [Elements of psychophysics]. Leipzig, Germany: Breitkopf & Hartel.

Finney, D. J. (1952). *Probit analysis: A statistical treatment of the sigmoid response curve,* 2nd ed. London: Cambridge University Press.

Fischer, G. H. (1997). Unidimensional linear logistic Rasch models. In W.J. van der Linden & R.K. Hambleton (Eds.), *Handbook of Modern Item Response theory* (pp. 225–243). New York: Springer-Verlag.

Fisher, R. A. (1922). On the mathematical foundations of theoretical statistics. *Proceedings of the Royal Society, 222*, 309–368.

Fisher, R. A. (1924). The conditions under which χ^2 measures the discrepancy between observations and hypothesis. *Journal of the Royal Statistical Society, 87*, 442–450.

Fisher, R. A. (1925). Theory of statistical estimation. *Proceedings of the Cambridge Philosophical Society, 22*, 699–725.

Fischer, G. H. (1977). Unidimensional linear logistic Rasch models. In W. J. van der Linder & R. K. Hambleton (Eds.), *Handbook of modern item response theory* (pp. 225–243). New York: Springer.

Garner, M. L. (1998) *Rasch measurement theory, the method of paired comparisons, and graph theory* (Unpublished doctoral dissertation). Emory University, Atlanta, Georgia. Retrieved December 6, 2008, from Dissertations & Theses @ Emory University database. (Publication No. AAT 9830147).

Garner, M., & Engelhard, G. (2000). Rasch measurement theory: The method of paired comparisons and graph theory. In M. Wilson & G. Engelhard (Eds.), *Objective measurement: Theory into practice, volume 5* (pp. 259–286). Stamford, CT: Ablex.

Garner, M., & Engelhard, G. (2002). An eigenvector method for estimating item parameters of the dichotomous and polytomous Rasch models. *Journal of Applied Measurement, 3*(2), 107–128.

Garner, M., & Engelhard, G. (2009). Using paired comparison matrices to estimate parameters of the partial credit Rasch measurement model for rater-mediated assessments. *Journal of Applied Measurement, 10*(1), 30–41.

Garner, M., & Engelhard, G. (2010). Extension of the pairwise algorithm to the rating scale and partial credit models. In M. Garner, G. Engelhard, M. Wilson, & W. Fisher (Eds.). *Advances in Rasch measurement, volume one* (pp. 45–63). Maple Grove, MN: JAM Press.

Goodenough, W.H. (1944). A technique for scale analysis. *Educational and Psychological Measurement, 4*, 179–190.

Goodman, L. A. (1975). A new model for scaling response patterns: An application of the quasi-independence concept. *Journal of the American Statistical Association, 70*, 755–768.

Guilford, J. P. (1936). *Psychometric methods.* New York: McGraw Hill.

Gulliksen, H. (1950). *Theory of mental tests.* New York: Wiley.

Guttman, L. (1944). A basis for scaling qualitative data. *American Sociological Review, 9*(2), 139–150.

Guttman, L. (1950). The basis for scalogram analysis. In S. A. Stouffer, L. Guttman, E. A. Suchman, P. F. Lazarsfeld, S. A. Star, & J. A. Clausen (Eds.), *Measurement and prediction* (Vol. IV, pp. 60–90). Princeton, NJ: Princeton University Press.

Guskey, T. R. (2006). Taxonomy of educational objectives, handbook I: The cognitive domain. In T. R.Guskey (Ed.), *Benjamin S. Bloom: Portraits of an educator* (pp. 38–44). Lanham, MD: Rowman & Littlefield Education.

Gyagenda, I. S., & Engelhard, G. (2009). Using classical and modern measurement theories to explore rater, domain, and gender Influences on student writing ability. *Journal of Applied Measurement, 10*(3), 225–246.

Gyagenda, I. S., & Engelhard, G. (2010). Rater, domain, and gender influences on the assessed quality of student writing. In Garner, M., Engelhard, G., Wilson, & M., Fisher, W. (Eds.), *Advances in Rasch measurement, volume one* (pp. 398–429). Maple Grove, MN: JAM Press.

Haberman, S. (1977). Maximum likelihood estimates in exponential response models. *The Annals of Statistics, 5*, 815–841.

Haberman, S. J. (2009).*Use of generalized residuals to examine goodness of fit of item response models* (ETS RR-09-15). Princeton, NJ: Educational Testing Service.

Haberman, S. J. (2009). *Use of generalized residuals to examine goodness of fit of item response models* (ETS RR-09-15). Princeton, NJ: Educational Testing Service.

Haley, D. C. (1952). Estimation of the dosage mortality relationship when the dose is subject to error. *Technical Report No. 15*, August 29, 1952. Stanford, CA: Contract No ONR-25140, Applied Mathematics and Statistics Laboratory, Stanford University.

Hambleton, R. K., & Han, N. (2005). Assessing the fit of IRT models to educational and psychological test data: A five step plan and several graphical displays. In W. R. Lenderking & D. Revicki (Eds.), *Advances in health outcomes research methods, measurement, statistical analysis, and clinical applications* (pp. 57–78). Washington, DC: Degnon Associates.

Hambleton, R. K., & Jones, R. W. (1993). Comparison of classical test theory and item response theory and their applications to test development. *Educational measurement: Issues and practice*, (Fall), 38–47.

Hammond, K. R. (1996). *Human judgment and social policy: Irreducible uncertainty, inevitable error, unavoidable injustice.* New York: Oxford University Press.

Hammond, K. R., & Stewart, T. R. (Eds.). (2001). *The essential Brunswik: Beginnings, explications, applications.* New York: Oxford University Press.

Hattie, J. (1985). Methodology review: Assessing unidimensionality of tests and items. *Applied Psychological Measurement, 9*(2), 139–164.

Hattie, J., Jaeger, R. M., & Bond, L. (1999). Persistent methodological questions in educational testing. In A. Iran-Nejad & P. D. Pearson (Eds.), *Review of research in education, 24*, 393–446. Thousand Oaks, CA: Sage.

Hedges, L. V., & Olkin, I. (1985). *Statistical methods for meta-analysis.* San Diego, CA: Academic Press.

Heinen, T. (1996). *Latent class and discrete latent trait models.* Thousand Oaks, CA: Sage Publications.

Hillegas, M. B. (1912). *A scale for the measurement of quality in English composition by young people.* New York: Teachers College, Columbia University.

Hogarth, R. (1987). *Judgment and choice: The psychology of decisions. Second edition.* New York: Wiley.

Hoyt, C .J. (1941). Test reliability estimated by analysis of variance. *Psychometrika, 6*, 153–160.

Hoyt, W. T. (2000). Rater bias in psychological research: When is it a problem and what can we do about it? *Psychological Methods, 5*(1), 64–86.

Hoyt, W. T., & Kerns, M. D. (1999). Magnitude and moderators of bias in observer ratings: A meta-analysis. *Psychological Methods, 4*(4), 403–424.

Huff, K., Steinberg, L., & Matts, T. (2010). The promises and challenges of implementing evidence-centered design in large-scale assessment. *Applied Measurement in Education, 23*(4), 310–324.

Huot, B. (1990). The literature of direct writing assessment: Major concerns and prevailing trends. *Review of Educational Research, 60*(2), 237–263.

Huynh, H. (1994). On equivalence between a partial credit item and a set of independent Rasch binary items. *Psychometrika, 59*, 111–119.

Huynh, H. (1996). Decomposition of a Rasch partial credit item into independent binary and indecomposable trinary items. *Psychometrika, 61*, 31–39.

Isaacson, W. (2007). *Einstein: His life and universe.* New York: Simon & Shuster.

Johnson, R. L., Penny, J. A., & Gordon, B. (2009). *Assessing performance: Designing, scoring, and validating performance tasks.* New York: Guilford Press.

Johnstone, C., Altman, J., & Thurlow, M. (2006). *A state guide to the development of universally designed assessments.* Minneapolis: University of Minnesota, National Center on Educational Outcomes.

Jaeger, R. M. (1987). Two decades of revolution in educational measurement!? *Educational Measurement: Issues and Practice, 6*, 6–14.

Jones, A. B. (2007). *Examining rater accuracy within the context of a high-stakes writing assessment* (Unpublished doctoral dissertation). Emory University, Atlanta, GA.

Joreskog, K. G. (1969). A general approach to confirmatory maximum likelihood factor analysis. *Psychometrika, 34*, 183–202.

Joreskog, K. G. (1971). Statistical analysis of sets of congeneric tests. Psychometrika, 36(2) 109–133.

Joreskog, K. G. (1974). Analyzing psychological data by structural analysis of covariance matrices. In D. H. Krantz, R. C. Atkinson, R. D. Luce, & P. Suppes (Eds.), *Contemporary developments in mathematical psychology* (Vol. 2, pp. 1–56). San Francisco: W.H. Freeman.

Joreskog, K. G. (2007). Factor analysis and its extensions. In R. Cudeck & R.C. MacCallum (Eds.), *Factor analysis at 100: Historical developments and future directions* (pp. 47–77). Mahwah, NJ: Erlbaum.

Kane, M. T. (2006). An argument-based approach to validation. *Psychological Bulletin, 112*, 527–535.

Karabatsos, G. (2000). A critique of Rasch residual fit statistics. *Journal of Applied Measurement, 1*(2), 152–176.

Kelderman, H. (1984). Loglinear Rasch model tests. *Psychometrika*, 49, 223–245.

Kendall, M. G., & Buckland, W. R. (1957). *Dictionary of statistical terms.* Edinburgh, Scotland: Oliver and Boyd.

Kolen, M. J., & Brennan, R. L. (2004).*Test equating, linking and scaling: Methods and practices, 2nd edition.* New York: Spring-Verlag.

Krathwohl, D. R., Bloom, B. S., & Masia, B. B. (1964). *Taxonomy of educational objectives, the classification of educational goals: Handbook II: The affective domain.* New York: McKay.

Kuder, G. F., & Richardson, M. W. (1937) The theory of estimation of test reliability. *Psychometrika, 2*, 151–160.

Kuhn, T. S. (1970). *The structure of scientific revolutions* (2nd ed.). Princeton, NJ: Princeton University Press.

Lakatos, I. (1978). *The methodology of scientific research programs.* Cambridge, UK: Cambridge University Press.

Lancaster, H. O. (1969). *The chi-squared distribution.* New York: Wiley.

Landy, F. J., & Farr, J. L. (1983). *The measurement of work performance: Methods, theory and applications.* New York: Academic Press.

Lane, S., & Stone, C. (2006). Performance assessment. In R. Brennan (Ed.), *Educational measurement, fourth edition* (pp. 387–431). Westport, CT: American Council on Education and Praeger.

Laudan, L. (1977). *Progress and its problems: Toward a theory of scientific change.* Berkeley: University of California Press.

Laudan, L. (1990). The history and the philosophy of science. In R. C. Olby et al. (Eds.), *Companion to the history of science* (pp. 47–59). London: Routledge.

Lawley, D. N. (1943). On problems connected with item selection and test construction. *Proceedings of the Royal Society of Edinburgh, 61,* 273–287.

Lazarsfeld, P. F. (1950a). The logical and mathematical foundation of latent structure analysis. In S. A. Stouffer, L. Guttman, E. A. Suchman, P. F. Lazarsfeld, S. A. Star, & J. A. Clausen (Eds.), *Measurement and prediction* (pp. 362–412). Princeton, NJ: Princeton University of Press.

Lazarsfeld, P. F. (1950b). The interpretation and computation of some latent structures. In S. A. Stouffer, L. Guttman, E. A. Suchman, P .F. Lazarsfeld, S. A. Star, & J. A. Clausen (Eds.), *Measurement and prediction* (pp. 413–472). Princeton, NJ: Princeton University of Press.

Lazarsfeld, P. F. (1958). Evidence and inference in social research. In D. Lerner (Ed.), *Evidence and inference* (pp. 107–138). Glencoe, IL: The Free Press.

Lazarsfeld, P. F. (1959). Latent structure analysis. In S. Koch (Ed.), *Psychology: A study of a science, Volume 3: Formulation of the person and the social context* (pp. 476–543). New York: McGraw-Hill.

Lazarsfeld, P. F. (1961). The algebra of dichotomous systems. H. Solomon (Ed.), *Studies in item analysis and prediction* (pp. 111–157). Stanford, CA: Stanford University Press.

Lazarsfeld, P. (1966). Concept formation and measurement in the behavioral sciences: Some historical observations. In G. J. Direnzo (Ed.), *Concepts, theory, and explanation in the behavioral sciences* (pp. 144–202). New York: Random House.

Lazarsfeld, P. F., & Henry, N. W. (1968). *Latent structure analysis.* Boston: Houghton-Mifflin.

Lewis, D. M., Mitzel, H. C., & Green, D. R. (1996, June). Standard setting: A Bookmark approach. In D. R. Green (Chair), *IRT-based standard setting procedures utilizing behavioral anchoring.* Symposium conducted at the meeting of the Council of Chief State School Officers National Conference on Large Scale Assessment, Phoenix, AZ.

Likert, R. (1932). A technique for the measurement of attitudes. *Archives of Psychology, 20*(140).

Linacre, J. M. (1989). *Many-facet Rasch measurement.* Chicago: MESA Press.

Linacre, J. M. (1994). *Many-facet Rasch measurement, 2nd ed.* Chicago: MESA Press.

Linacre, J. M. (1999). Investigating rating scale category usage. *Journal of Outcome Measurement, 3*(2), 103–122.

Linacre, J. M. (2004a). Estimation methods for Rasch measures. In In E. V. Smith & R. M. Smith (Eds.), *Introduction to Rasch measurement: Theory, models, and applications* (pp. 25–47). Maple Grove, MN: JAM Press.

Linacre, J. M. (2004b). Rasch model estimation: Further topics. In E. V. Smith & R.

M. Smith (Eds.), *Introduction to Rasch measurement: Theory, models, and applications* (pp. 48–72). Maple Grove, MN: JAM Press.

Linacre, J. M. (2007). *A user's guide to FACETS: Rasch-model computer programs.* Retrieved from www.winsteps.com.

Linn, R. L., Gronlund, N. E., & Miller, M. D. (2008). *Measurement and assessment in teaching, 10th ed.* New York: Prentice Hall.

Lloyd-Jones, R. (1977). Primary trait scoring. In C. R. Cooper & L. Odell (Eds.), *Evaluating writing* (pp. 33–69). New York: National Council of Teachers of English.

Loevinger, J. (1965). Person and population as psychometric concepts. *Psychological Review, 72*, 143–155.

Lord, F. M. (1952). A theory of test scores. *Psychometric Monograph. No. 7.*

Lord, F. M. (1980). Applications of item response theory to practical testing problems. Hillsdale, NJ: Erlbaum.

Lord, F. M., & Novick, M. R. (1968). Statistical theories of mental test scores. Reading, MA: Addison-Wesley.

Luecht, R. M. (1998). Computer assisted test assembly using optimization heuristics. *Applied Psychological Measurement, 22,* 224–236.

Lumsden, J. (1977). Person reliability. *Applied Psychological Measurement, 1*(4), 477–482.

Masters, G. N. (1982). A Rasch model for partial credit scoring. *Psychometrika, 47,* 149–174.

Masters, G. N., & Wright, B. D. (1997). The partial credit model. In W. J. van der Linder & R. K. Hambleton (Eds.), *Handbook of modern item response theory* (pp. 101–121). New York: Springer.

Masters, G. N., & Wright, B. D. (1984). The essential process in a family of measurement models. *Psychometrika, 49,* 529–544.

McDonald, R. (1985). *Factor analysis and related methods.* Hillsdal, NJ: Erlbaum.

McNamara, T. F. (1996). *Measuring second language performance.* London: Longman.

Meredith, W. (1993). Measurement invariance, factor analysis, and factorial invariance. *Psychometrika, 58,* 525–543.

Messick, S. (1983). Assessment of children. In P. H. Mussen (Ed.), *Handbook of child psychology, volume 1: History, theory and methods* (pp. 477–526). New York: Wiley.

Messick, S. (1989). Validity. In R. Linn (Ed.), *Educational measurement, third edition* (pp. 13–103). Washington, DC: American Council on Education.

Millsap, R. E. (2011). *Statistical approaches to measurement invariance.* New York: Routledge.

Millsap, R. E. (2007). Invariance in measurement and prediction revisited. *Psychometrika, 72* (4), 461–473.

Millsap, R. E., & Meredith, W. (2007). Factorial invariance: Historical perspectives and new problems. In R. Cudeck & R. C. MacCallum (Eds.), *Factor analysis at 100: Historical developments and future directions* (pp. 131–152). Mahwah, NJ: Erlbaum.

Mislevy, R. J., & Bock, R. D. (1982). Biweight estimates of latent ability. *Educational and Psychological Measurement, 42,* 725–737.

Mislevy, R. J., & Haertel, G. D. (2006). Implications of evidence-centered design for educational testing. *Educational Measurement: Issues and Practice*, (Winter), 6–20.

Mislevy, R. J., Steinberg, L.S., Breyer, F. J., Almond, R. G., & Johnson, L. (2002). Making sense of data from complex assessments. *Applied Measurement in Education, 15*(4), 363–389.

Mitzel, H. C., Lewis, D. M., Patz, R. J., & Green, D. R. (2001). The bookmark procedure: Psychological perspectives. In G. J. Cizek (Ed.), *Setting performance standards: Concepts, methods and perspectives* (pp. 249–281). Mahwah, NJ: Erlbaum.

Mokken, R. J. (1971). *A theory and procedure of scale analysis.* The Hague: Mouton/ Berlin: De Gruyter.

Mokken, R. J. (1997). Nonparametric models for dichotomous responses. In W. J. van der Linden & R. K. Hambleton (Eds.), *Handbook of modern item response theory* (pp. 351–367). New York: Springer-Verlag.

Molenaar, I .W. (1997). Nonparametric models for polytomous responses. In W. J. van der Linder & R. K . Hambleton (Eds.), *Handbook of modern item response theory* (pp. 369–380). New York: Springer.

Monmonmier, M. (1996). *How to lie with maps.* Chicago: The University of Chicago Press.

Monsaas, J. A., & Engelhard, G. (1996). Examining changes in the home environment with the Rasch measurement model. In G. Engelhard, & M. Wilson (Eds.), *Objective measurement: Theory into practice, Volume 3* (pp. 127–140). Norwood, NJ: Ablex.

Mosier, C. I. (1940). Psychophysics and mental test theory: Fundamental postulates and elementary theorems. *Psychological Review, 47,* 355–366.

Mosier, C. I. (1941). Psychophysics and mental test theory II: The constant process *Psychological Review, 48,* 235–249.

Mulaik, S. A. (1986). Factor analysis and Psychometrika: Major developments. *Psychometrika, 51*(1), 23–33.

Muraki, E. (1990). Fitting a polytomous item response model to Likert-type data. *Applied Psychological Measurement, 14,* 59–71.

Muraki, E. (1992). A generalized partial credit model. Application of an EM algorithm. *Applied Psychological Measurement, 16,* 159–176.

Muraki, E. (1997). A generalized partial credit model. In W. J. van der Linder & R. K. Hambleton (Eds.), *Handbook of modern item response theory* (pp. 153–164). New York: Springer.

Muraki, E., & Engelhard, G. (1985). Full-information item factor analysis: Applications of EAP scores. *Applied Psychological Measurement, 9*(4), 417–430.

Murphy, K. R., & Cleveland, J. N. (1995). *Understanding performance appraisal: Social, organizational, and goal-based perspectives.* Thousand Oaks, CA: Sage.

Myford, C. M., & Wolfe, E. W. (2003). Detecting and measuring rater effects using many-facet Rasch measurement: Part I. *Journal of Applied Measurement, 4,* 386–422.

Myford, C. M., & Wolfe, E. W. (2004). Detecting and measuring rater effects using many-facet Rasch measurement: Part II. *Journal of Educational Measurement, 46,* 371–389.

Myford, C. M., & Wolfe, E. W. (2009). Monitoring rater performance over time: A framework for detecting differential accuracy and differential scale category use. *Journal of Applied Measurement, 5,* 189–227.

Nunnally, J. C. (1967). *Psychometric theory.* New York: McGraw-Hill Book Company.

Pearson, K. (1900). On the criterion that a given system of deviations from the probable in the case of a correlated system of variables is such that it can be reasonably supposed to have arisen from random sampling. *Philosophy Magazine, 50,* 157–172.

Perkins, A., & Engelhard, G. (2009). Crossing person response functions. *Rasch Measurement Transaction, 23*(1), 1183–1184.

Plackett, R. L. (1983). Karl Pearson and the chi-squared test. *International Statistical Review, 51*(1), 59–72.

Popper, K. (1959). *The logic of scientific discovery* (translation of Logik der Forschung). London: Hutchinson.

Popper, K. (1963). *Conjectures and refutations: The growth of scientific knowledge.* London: Routledge.

Porter, T. M. (1986). *The rise of statistical thinking, 1820–1900.* Princeton, NJ: Princeton University Press.

Porter, T. M. (1995). *Trust in numbers: The pursuit of objectivity in science and public life.* Princeton, NJ: Princeton University Press.

Porter, T. M. (2003). Measurement, objectivity, and trust. *Measurement: Interdisciplinary Research and Perspectives, 1*(4), 241–255.

Postman, L., & Tolman, E. C. (1959). Brunswik's probabilistic functionalism. In S. Koch (Ed.), *Psychology: A study of a science* (pp. 502–564). New York: McGraw-Hill.

Ramsay, J. O., & Silverman, B. W. (2002). *Applied functional data analysis: Methods and case studies.* New York: Springer-Verlag.

Randall, J., & Engelhard, G. (2009). Examining teacher grades using Rasch measurement theory. *Journal of Educational Measurement, 46*(1) 1–18.

Randall, J. D. (2007). *Using Guttman's facet theory to examine the grading practices of teachers* (Unpublished doctoral dissertation). Emory University. Atlanta, GA. Dissertation Abstracts International, Volume: 68–05, Section: A, page: 1902.

Rasch, G. (1960/1980). *Probabilistic models for some intelligence and attainment tests.* Copenhagen: Danish Institute for Educational Research. (Expanded edition, Chicago: University of Chicago Press, 1980).

Rasch, G. (1961). On general laws and meaning of measurement in psychology. In J. Neyman (Ed.), *Proceedings of the fourth Berkeley Symposium on mathematical statistics and probability* (pp. 321–333). Berkeley: University of California Press.

Rasch, G. (1977). On specific objectivity: An attempt at formalizing the request for generality and validity of scientific statements. *Danish Yearbook of Philosophy, 14,* 58–94.

Raudenbush, S. W., & Bryk, A. S. (2002). *Hierarchical linear models: Applications and data analysis methods* (2nd ed.) Thousand Oaks, CA: Sage.

Read, T. R. C., & Cressie, N. A. C. (1988). *Goodness-of-fit for discrete multivariate data.* New York: Springer-Verlag.

Reckase, M. D. (1979). Unifactor latent trait models applied to multifactor tests: Results and implications. *Journal of Educational Statistics, 4,* 207–230.

Reckase, M. D. (2009). *Multidimensional item response theory.* New York: Springer.

Richardson, M. W. (1936). The relationship between item difficulty and the differential validity of a test. *Psychometrika, 1,* 33–49.

Ryan, D. D. (2007). *Measurement of student nurse performance in the safe administra-*

tion of medication (Unpublished doctoral dissertation). Emory University, Atlanta, GA. Dissertation Abstracts International, Volume: 68–09, Section: A, page: 3819.

Saal, F. E., Downey, R. G., & Lahey, M. A. (1980). Rating the ratings: Assessing the psychometric quality rating data. *Psychological Bulletin, 88*(2), 413–428.

Samejima, F. (1969). Estimation of latent ability using a response pattern of graded scores. *Psychometrika Monograph,* No. 17.

Samejima, F. (1983). Some methods and approaches for estimating the operating characteristics of discrete item responses. In H. Wainer & S. Messick (Eds.), *Principle of modern psychological measurement: A festschrift for Frederic M. Lord* (pp. 159–182). Hillsdale, NJ: Erlbaum.

Samejima, F. (1997). The graded response model. In W. J. van der Linder & R. K. Hambleton (Eds.), *Handbook of modern item response theory* (pp. 85–100). New York: Springer.

Schmeiser, C. B., & Welch, C. J. (2006). Test development. In R. L. Brennan (Ed.), *Educational measurement, 4th edition* (pp. 307–353). Westport, CT: Praeger.

Shewhart, W. A. (1939). *Statistical method from the viewpoint of quality control.* Lancaster, PA: The Lancaster Press.

Shrout, P. E., & Fleiss, J. L. (1979). Intraclass correlations: Uses in assessing rater reliability. *Psychological Bulletin, 86* (2), 420–428.

Siegel, S. (1956). *Nonparametric statistics for the behavioral sciences.* New York: McGraw-Hill Book Company.

Sijtsma, K., & Meijer, R.R. (2007). Nonparametric item response theory and special topics. In C.R. Rao & S. Sinharay (Eds.), *Psychometrics, handbook of statistics* (Vol. 26, pp. 719–747). Amsterdam: Elsevier.

Sijtsma, K. A., & Molenaar, I. W. (2002). *Introduction to nonparametric item response theory.* Thousand Oaks, CA: Sage.

Smith, R. M. (2004). Fit analysis in latent trait measurement models. In E. V. Smith & R. M. Smith (Eds.), *Introduction to Rasch measurement: Theory, models and applications* (pp. 73–91). Maple Grove, MN: JAM Press.

Smith, R. M., & Hedges, L. V. (1982). A comparison of likelihood ratio χ^2 and Pearsonian χ^2 tests of fit in the Rasch model. *Educational Research and Perspectives, 9*, 44–54.

Spearman, C. (1904a). "General intelligence," objectively determined and measured. *American Journal of Psychology, 15*, 201–293.

Spearman, C. (1904b). The proof and measurement of association between two things. *American Journal of Psychology, 15*, 72–101.

Spearman, C. (1907). Demonstration of formulae for true measurement of correlation. *American Journal of Psychology, 18*, 160–169.

Spearman, C. (1910). Correlation calculated from faulty data. *British Journal of Psychology, 3*, 271–295.

Spearman, C. (1927). *The abilities of man: Their nature and measurement.* New York: Macmillan.

Stevens, S.S. (1946). On the theory of scales of measurement. *Science 103*(2684), 677–680.

Stevens, S. S. (1951). Mathematics, measurement and psychophysics. In S .S. Stevens (Ed.), *Handbook of experimental psychology* (pp. 1–49). New York: Wiley.

Stallings, W. M., & Gillmore, G. M. (1971). A note on "accuracy" and "precision." *Journal of Educational Measurement, 8*(2), 127–129.

Still, A. (1987). L.L. Thurstone: A new assessment. *British Journal of Mathematical and Statistical Psychology, 40*, 101–108.

Stone, M. H., Wright, B. D., & Stenner, J. A. (1999). Mapping variables. *Journal of Outcome Measurement, 3*(4), 308–322.

Stouffer, S. A., Guttman, L., Suchman, E. A., Lazarsfeld, P. F., Star, S. A., & Clausen, J. A. (1950). *Measurement and prediction* (Vol. IV). Princeton, NJ: Princeton University Press.

Sulsky, L. M., & Balzer, W. K. (1988). Meaning and measurement of performance rating accuracy: Some methodological and theoretical concerns. *Journal of Applied Psychology, 73*, 497–506.

Stouffer, S. A., & Toby, J. (1951). Role conflict and personality. *The American Journal of Sociology, 56*, 395–406.

Swaminathan, H., & Gifford, J. A. (1982). Bayesian estimation in the Rasch model. *Journal of Educational Statistics, 7*, 175–191.

Swaminathan, H., Hambleton, R. K., & Rogers, H. J. (2007). Assessing the fit of item response theory models (pp. 683–718). In C. R. Rao & S. Sinharay (Eds.), *Psychometrics, handbook of statistics* (Vol. 26, pp. 683–718). Amsterdam: Elsevier.

Thissen, D. (1982). Marginal maximum likelihood estimation for the one-parameter logistic model. *Psychometrika, 47*, 175–186.

Thissen, D., & Steinberg, L. (1986). A taxonomy of item response models. *Psychometrika, 51*(4), 567–577.

Thorndike, E. L. (1904). *An introduction to the theory of mental and social measurements.* New York: Teachers College, Columbia University.

Thorndike, E. L. (1913). Educational measurements of fifty years ago. *Journal of Educational Psychology, 6*, 551–552.

Thorndike, E. L. (1914). The measurement of ability in reading. *Teachers College Record, 15*(4), 207–277.

Thorndike, E. L. (1916). *English composition: 150 Specimens arranged for use in psychological and educational experiments.* New York: Teachers College, Columbia University.

Thorndike, E. L. (1919). *An introduction to the theory of mental and social measurements.* New York: Teachers College Press.

Thorndike, E. L. (1920). A constant error in psychological ratings. *Journal of Applied Psychology, 4*, 25–29.

Thorndike, E. L. (1945). Charles Edward Spearman: 1863–1945. *The American Journal of Psychology, LVIII*, 558–560.

Thurlow, M. L., Quenemoen, R. F., Lazarus, S. S., Moen, R. E., Johnstone, C. J., Liu, K., et al. (2008). *A principled approach to accountability assessments for students with disabilities* (Synthesis Report 70). Minneapolis: University of Minnesota, National Center on Educational Outcomes.

Thurstone, L. L. (1925). A method of scaling psychological and educational tests. *Journal of Educational Psychology, 16*, 433–451.

Thurstone, L. L. (1926). The scoring of individual performance. *Journal of Educational Psychology, 17*, 446–457.

Thurstone, L. L. (1927). The method of paired comparisons for social values. *Journal of Abnormal and Social Psychology, 21*, 384–400.

Thurstone, L. L. (1928, July-October). Experimental study of nationality preferences. *Journal of General Psychology*, 405–205.

Thurstone, L. L. (1931). *The reliability and validity of tests.* Ann Arbor, MI: Edwards.

Thurstone, L. L. (1935). *The vectors of mind.* Chicago: University of Chicago Press.

Thurstone, L .L. (19947). *Multiple factor analysis.* Chicago: University of Chicago Press.

Thurstone, L. L. (1952). Autobiography. In E. G. Boring, H. S. Langfield, H. Werner, & R. M. Uerkes (Eds.), *A history of psychology in autobiography, Vol. 4* (pp. 295–321). Worcester, MA: Clark University Press.

Thurstone, L. L. (1959). *The measurement of values.* Chicago: The University of Chicago Press.

Thurstone, L. L., & Chave, E. J. (1929). *The measurement of attitude: A psychophysical method and some experiments for measuring attitude toward the church.* Chicago: The University of Chicago Press.

Toksika, V., & Sylva, K. (2004). The home observation for measurement of the environment revisited. *Child and Adolescent Mental Health, 9*(1), 25–35.

Torgerson, W. S. (1958). *Theory and methods of scaling.* New York: Wiley.

Trabue, M. R. (1916). *Completion-test language scales.* New York: Teachers College, Columbia University.

Trabin, T. E., & Weiss, D. J. (1983). The person response curve: Fit of individuals to item response theory models. In D. J. Weiss (Ed.), *New horizons in testing: Latent trait test theory and computerized adaptive testing* (pp. 83–108). New York: Academic Press.

Traub, R. (1997). Classical test theory in historical perspective. *Educational Measurement: Issues and practice, 16*(10), 8–13.

Urban, F. M. (1908). *The application of statistical methods to the problems of psychophysics.* Philadelphia: Psychological Clinic Press.

van der Linden, W. J., & Hambleton, R. K. (Eds.). (1997). *Handbook of modern item response theory.* New York: Springer.

Verhelst, N. D., & Glas, C. A. W. (1995). The one parameter logistic model. In G. H. Fischer & I. W. Molenaar (Eds.), *Rasch models: Foundations, recent developments, and applications* (pp. 215–237). New York: Springer Verlag.

Vogel, S. P., & Engelhard, G. (2011). Using Rasch Measurement Theory to Examine Two Instructional Approaches for Teaching and Learning of French Grammar. *Journal of Educational Research, 104,* 267–282.

von Eye, A., & Mun, E. Y. (2005). *Analyzing rater agreement: Manifest variable methods.* Mahwah, NJ: Erlbaum.

Warm, T. A. (1989). Weighted likelihood estimation of ability in item response theory. *Psychometrika, 54*(23), 427–450.

Wainer, H., & Wright, B. D. (1980). Robust estimation of ability in the Rasch model. *Psychometrika, 45,* 373–391.

Wherry, R. J. (1952). *The control of bias in rating: A theory of rating.* (Personnel Research Report 922). Washington, DC: Department of the Army, Personnel Research Section.

Wiggins, G. (1989). A true test: Toward more authentic and equitable assessment. *Phi Delta Kappan, 79,* 703–713.

Wilks, S. S. (1935). The likelihood test of independence in contingency tables. *Annals of Mathematical Statistics, 6,* 190–196.

Wilson, M. (2005). *Constructing measures: An item response modeling approach (2nd edition).* Mahwah, NJ: Erlbaum.

Wind, S. A., & Engelhard, G. (2011, July). *Evaluating the quality of ratings in writing assessment: Rater agreement, precision, and accuracy.* Paper presented at the Pacific Rim Objective Measurement Seminar (PROMS) in Singapore.

Wolfe, E. W., Myford, C. M., Engelhard, G., & Manalo, J. R. (2007). *Monitoring reader performance and DRIFT in the AP English Literature and Composition Examination using benchmark essays.* New York: The College Board.

Woody, C. (1920). *Measurements of some achievements in arithmetic.* New York: Teachers College, Columbia University.

Wright, B. D. (1968). Sample-free test calibration and person measurement. In *Proceedings of the 1967 invitational conference on testing problems* (pp. 85–101). Princeton, NJ: Educational Testing Service.

Wright, B. D. (1977). Solving measurement problems with the Rasch model. *Journal of Educational Measurement, 14*(2), 97–116.

Wright, B. D. (1980). Afterward. In G. Rasch (1960/1980), *Probabilistic models for some intelligence and attainment tests* (pp. 185–194). Copenhagen: Danish Institute for Educational Research. (Expanded edition, Chicago: University of Chicago Press, 1980).

Wright, B. D. (1993). Logits? *Rasch measurement transactions, 7*(2), 288.

Wright, B. D. (1997, Winter). A history of social science measurement. *Educational Measurement: Issues and Practice*, 33– 45, 52.

Wright, B. D., & Masters, G. N. (1982). *Rating scale analysis: Rasch measurement.* Chicago: MESA Press.

Wright, B. D., & Panchapakesan, N. (1969). A procedure for sample-free item analysis. *Educational and Psychological Measurement, 29*, 23–48.

Wright, B. D., & Stone, M. (1979). *Best test design: Rasch measurement.* Chicago: MESA Press.

Wu, M. L., Adams, R. J., & Wilson, M. R. (1997). *ConQuest: Generalised item response modeling software.* Melbourne, Australia: ACER.

Yanai, H. & Kchikawa, M. (2007). Factor analysis. In C.R. Rao and S. Sinharay (Eds.). *Psychometrics, handbook of statistics* (Vol. 26, pp. 257–296). Amsterdam: Elsevier.

Yuan, K., & Bentler, P. M. (2007). Structural equation modeling. In C. R. Rao & S. Sinharay (Eds.), *Psychometrics, handbook of statistics* (Vol. 6, pp. 297–358). Amsterdam: Elsevier.

Zucker, S., Sassman, C., & Case, B. J. (2004). *Cognitive labs.* San Antonio, TX: Pearson Education.

Zumbo, B. D. (1999). *A handbook on the theory and methods of differential item functioning (DIF): Logistic regression modeling as a unitary framework for binary and Likert-type (ordinal) item scores.* Ottawa, ON: Directorate of Human Resources Research and Evaluation, Department of National Defense.

Author Index

Subject Index